T0181793

Understanding Military Workforce Productivity

Robert M. Bray • Laurel L. Hourani
Jason Williams • Marian E. Lane
Mary Ellen Marsden

Understanding Military Workforce Productivity

Effects of Substance Abuse, Health, and Mental Health

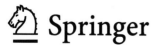 Springer

Robert M. Bray
RTI International
Research Triangle Park, NC, USA

Laurel L. Hourani
RTI International
Research Triangle Park, NC, USA

Jason Williams
RTI International
Research Triangle Park, NC, USA

Marian E. Lane
RTI International
Research Triangle Park, NC, USA

Mary Ellen Marsden
RTI International
Research Triangle Park, NC, USA

ISBN 978-1-4939-5055-3   ISBN 978-0-387-78303-1 (eBook)
DOI 10.1007/978-0-387-78303-1
Springer New York Heidelberg Dordrecht London

Preface

Our military men and women are regularly called upon to defend and support United States' interests across the world in combat and noncombat situations. These demands call for a highly functioning, productive force that is ready and able to respond to military requirements on short notice. This book examines challenges faced by service members and the conditions that affect their ability to respond to the multiple demands placed upon them. The challenges are many—recurring deployments, combat experiences, separation from home and family, the risk of injury or death, and problems in reintegration. How these challenges are met affects force productivity and the readiness of service members to perform their military mission. Substance abuse, poor health behaviors, and mental health problems interact with these challenges and may result in lowered force productivity.

This book examines trends in substance abuse, health, and mental health of the active duty military and provides the first broad-based examination of their independent and combined effects on force productivity and readiness based on original analyses. One of the key contributions of our study is the assessment of the influence of an array of complex factors in these important cross-cutting domains. Information on these issues is drawn from a series of 10 comprehensive surveys conducted between 1980 and 2008 of the U.S. military population stationed across the world. Begun in 1980, the Department of Defense (DoD) Surveys of Health Related Behaviors Among Active Duty Military Personnel (referred to here as the HRB surveys) were conducted for DoD by RTI International (RTI) from 1982 to 2008. The surveys are unique in selecting samples that represent the active duty military population comprising personnel in the Army, Navy, Marine Corps, and Air Force and are widely recognized as the most comprehensive source of information about substance abuse, health, and mental health of the active duty force. The surveys have been used as a broad barometer of how health, mental health, and substance abuse programs are working and as a signal of where adjustments in programs and policies may be needed.

The purpose of this book is to identify the health and behavioral health challenges faced by military men and women and the policy and programmatic implications of these challenges. Findings will be useful for military officials, policymakers, and researchers interested in a better understanding of military force productivity and ways to improve it. Although the series of HRB surveys has described trends in substance abuse, health, and mental health of our force over 3 decades, in-depth modeling of these outcomes has not been previously reported and the impact of the independent and combined effects of these behaviors and conditions on military force productivity has not been documented.

The authors of this book have all contributed to the conduct of the HRB survey and related analyses over the past 3 decades, in partnership with DoD. The senior author, Robert M. Bray, led the HRB surveys from 1982 to 2008, while the other four authors—Laurel L. Hourani, Jason Williams, Marian E. Lane, and Mary Ellen Marsden—have been contributors to the design of the study, analyses, and writing of the study final reports and other scientific papers based on these data. Drs. Bray, Hourani, Williams, and Lane are staff members of RTI. Dr. Marsden, who recently retired from RTI, contributed significantly to conceptualizing and writing this book but was unable to see it to completion. Numerous additional staff at RTI have contributed to the survey over the years, and the analyses reported here draw on their contributions.

This book is dedicated to the service, courage, commitment, and sacrifices of our military men and women and to their families who have supported them.

Research Triangle Park, NC, USA

Robert M. Bray
Laurel L. Hourani
Jason Williams
Marian E. Lane
Mary Ellen Marsden

About the Authors

Robert M. Bray, Ph.D., a fellow of the American Psychological Association, is a Senior Research Psychologist and Senior Director of the Substance Abuse Epidemiology and Military Behavioral Health Program at RTI International. His research interests focus on the epidemiology of substance use and other health behaviors in military and civilian populations, with an emphasis on understanding the prevalence, causes, correlates, and consequences of these behaviors. He has directed nine comprehensive worldwide Department of Defense Surveys of Health Related Behaviors Among Active Duty Military Personnel, which have furnished the most widely cited data on substance use and health behaviors in the active duty military and which serve as the basis for the findings in this book. He has directed and/or supported other studies of the military population assessing health-related behaviors among the Reserve component, risk and protective factors for initiation of tobacco and alcohol use, mental fitness and resilience among Army basic combat trainees, and a Web-based intervention to reduce heavy alcohol use among active duty service members. He is currently leading the RTI International component of a large multi-institutional clinical trial to optimize usual primary care for soldiers with posttraumatic stress disorder and depression. Dr. Bray is principal editor of the book *Drug Use in Metropolitan America*, which integrates findings from a large-scale study of drug use among diverse populations in the Washington, DC, metropolitan area. He has published and presented widely in the area of substance use- and health-related behaviors. Dr. Bray received his Ph.D. in Social Psychology from the University of Illinois.

Laurel L. Hourani, Ph.D., M.P.H., joined RTI International in 2001 as a research epidemiologist after heading the Health Sciences Division of the Naval Health Research Center in San Diego. She has conducted health and psychological research in the United States and abroad for more than 20 years and has extensive experience with military populations. Dr. Hourani's expertise and main research interests are in the areas of mental health and substance abuse. She has been the principal investigator on several military-sponsored studies of suicide and mental disorders among the U.S. Navy and Marine Corps personnel and was instrumental in the development and annual analysis of the Department of the Navy Suicide Incident Report, which later became the basis for the current Department of Defense Suicide Event Report. She was associate project director for the 2002, 2005, and 2008 Department of Defense Surveys of Health Related Behaviors Among Active Duty Military Personnel and pioneered the Surveys of Health Related Behavior for the Reserve Component, both of which have served as models for military behavioral health research. She is currently leading a project on posttraumatic stress disorder that includes the development and testing of pre-deployment stress inoculation training programs in the Marine Corps and Army to prepare warriors psychologically to better deal with combat and operational stress. Dr. Hourani received her Ph.D. in Psychiatric Epidemiology from the University of Pittsburgh and is a Fellow of the American Psychological Association.

Jason Williams, Ph.D., is a Research Psychologist at RTI International with extensive experience in applying advanced statistical methods to the estimation and modeling of behavioral and mental health outcomes in military personnel. Dr. Williams has led the analyses for many large- and small-scale survey and program evaluation projects, including the Department of Defense Surveys of Health Related Behaviors Among Active Duty Military Personnel and the companion surveys for the Reserve Component. Dr. Williams' substantive research interests include program evaluation and substance use and violence prevention in at-risk populations such as youth and military personnel. In addition to leading analysis tasks for multiple studies, he conducts methodological development and applications studies, primarily in the area of mediation, including a National Institutes of Health-funded study examining methods of comparing mediated effects across groups. He has authored or coauthored multiple peer-reviewed articles on measurement of military-relevant mental health constructs such as PTSD as well as papers applying complex longitudinal and mediation models to military program evaluations and models of substance use. Dr. Williams received his Ph.D. in Social Psychology from Arizona State University.

Marian E. Lane, Ph.D., is a Research Psychologist at RTI International. She has more than 12 years of experience in industrial–organizational psychology, including more than a decade of studies of active duty and Reserve component personnel with an emphasis on substance abuse, mental health, and workforce productivity. At RTI, she has led numerous military research studies, including the Navy and Marine Corps Reservists Needs Assessment and the DoD/VA Integrated Mental Health Strategy (IMHS) Strategic Action #23: Chaplains' Roles studies. She has been a lead analyst for the Department of Defense Surveys of Health Related Behaviors Among Active Duty and Reserve Component Military Personnel. Her areas of expertise include survey research, multivariate statistics, focus group and key informant interviews, and organizational assessment, and she has had responsibility for study design, implementation, and evaluation of program effects. She has authored and coauthored articles on military mental health and substance abuse for peer-reviewed journals, presentations for national and international conferences, and briefings for senior military and civilian leaders. Dr. Lane received her Ph.D. in Experimental Psychology from the University of Memphis.

Mary Ellen Marsden, Ph.D., has more than 35 years of experience in the study of substance use epidemiology, treatment effectiveness, treatment organization, and policy issues. In her 20 years as a Senior Research Sociologist at RTI International, she was an analyst on eight Department of Defense Surveys of Health Related Behaviors Among Active Duty Military Personnel, reporting director for the National Survey on Drug Use and Health, and associate director of the National Analytic Center for the National Household Survey on Drug Abuse. She is coauthor of *Drug Abuse Treatment: A National Study of Effectiveness*, coeditor of *Drug Use in Metropolitan America*, and author of numerous articles on substance use among youth and military personnel, substance abuse treatment, and the substance abuse treatment system. Dr. Marsden received her Ph.D. in Sociology from the University of Chicago.

Acknowledgments

Many individuals made substantial contributions to the design and implementation of the Department of Defense Surveys of Health Related Behaviors Among Active Duty Military Personnel, which provided the data for this book. This book includes many original analyses from these surveys that were designed for this study and which appear here for the first time. First and foremost we acknowledge the contribution of each of the military men and women who responded to the surveys over the past 3 decades. Without the time they gave to answering a series of questions about their behaviors, the surveys—and this book—would not have been possible. In addition, we express our appreciation to the numerous military liaisons both at the headquarters of each military service and at the participating military installations (around 60 for each survey wave) for their dedication in ensuring coordination of complex field operations that made it possible to obtain the survey information.

We are indebted to the many individuals at the Department of Defense who have supported and guided the surveys over the years, dating back to the 1980s. Included in this group of Defense employees are current and former project officers for the surveys, current and former Assistant Secretaries of Defense for Health Affairs, and current and former Under Secretaries of Defense for Personnel and Readiness. We especially want to thank the individuals who assisted with the Department of Defense clearance process and provided comments on the draft manuscript.

In addition to the authors of this book, many other staff at RTI International made important contributions to the surveys. RTI staff who were major contributors to the 2008 Health Related Behavior survey, which forms the basis of many of the analyses discussed here, include Michael Pemberton, Michael Witt, Kristine Rae Olmsted, Janice Brown, BeLinda Weimer, Scott Scheffler, Russ Vandermaas-Peeler, Kimberly Aspinwall, Erin Anderson, Kathryn Spagnola, Kelly Close, Jennifer Gratton, Sara Calvin, and Michael Bradshaw. Their efforts covered designing the survey questionnaire, developing the sampling frame and selecting the sample of participants, directing and participating in survey teams that traveled to military installations worldwide to administer the questionnaires to service members, conducting statistical analyses, and writing and coauthoring the survey final technical report. For this book, special thanks go to Erin Anderson who coordinated reviews of the literature and figure production, to Shari Lambert, Valerie Garner, and Ally Elspas who produced the figures presented in the book, and to Justin Faerber who edited the volume.

We owe a debt of gratitude to RTI International for providing a positive and supportive working environment for us to think and to write and for a Professional Development award to Drs. Bray, Marsden, and Hourani that helped fund the preparation of this book. We express special thanks and appreciation to Dr. Gary Zarkin, Vice President of the Behavioral Health and Criminal Justice Division, Dr. Jan Mitchell, Vice President of the Social Policy, Health, & Economics Research Unit, Mr. Tim Gabel, Executive Vice President of Social, Statistical, and Environmental Sciences, and Dr. Wayne Holden, President and Chief Executive Officer for their encouragement of this project.

We also thank the staff at Springer for their interest in the book concept and their patience during the writing process. In particular, we acknowledge Bill Tucker, Editorial Director Behavioral Science, for his interest and help, and Khristine Queja and Christina Tuballes for their editorial assistance, oversight, and management of the production and publishing process.

Finally, we note that the views and opinions expressed in this book are solely those of the authors. They do not represent and should not be construed as an official policy or position of the U.S. Department of Defense, the branches of the U.S. military services, or the U.S. Government.

Research Triangle Park, NC, USA   Robert M. Bray
                                                                   Laurel L. Hourani
                                                                   Jason Williams
                                                                   Marian E. Lane
                                                                   Mary Ellen Marsden

Contents

Chapter 1
Health and Behavioral Health in the Military

1.1 Overview and Background

The U.S. military has spent over a decade in the longest and one of the most challenging sets of conflicts in our nation's history—the wars in Iraq and Afghanistan (2001 to the present, collectively). These conflicts have placed extensive stress and strain on military members from all service branches and on their families, including spouses, children, parents, and siblings. This is not surprising in view of the high operational tempo that has been in effect for an extended period and the frequent and lengthy large-scale deployments that have resulted in a combination of visible and invisible wounds of war in addition to loss of life. Even though Operation Iraqi Freedom (OIF) has officially concluded and Operation Enduring Freedom (OEF) is beginning to wind down, many of the substance abuse, physical health, and mental health concerns that emerged during the height and intensity of these conflicts are continuing issues for the military. The dynamics and sequelae of training, deploying, experiencing combat and combat-related traumas in theater, supporting others, and reintegrating after returning home are complex processes for service members and families to navigate (Adler, Bliese, & Castro, 2011; MacDermid Wadsworth & Riggs, 2011; Riviere & Merrill, 2011). Unfortunately, a sizable number of dedicated personnel experience physical health, mental health, and substance abuse problems stemming from their military experiences. Not only do these losses occur for service members and their families but they also diminish the ability of the military to provide continued high-level functioning of the active duty force and to meet the military mission. The costs of substance abuse, poor physical health, and mental health problems—whether they are monetary, legal, and/or personal/family-related—compromise our military's ability to protect the nation in the most effective, efficient manner.

To understand these complex issues, which impair military readiness and reduce military productivity, this book uses population-based data to examine these problems and their correlates across the military. This book is the first effort to provide a broad integrative look at the nature and extent of substance abuse, health status

R.M. Bray et al., *Understanding Military Workforce Productivity: Effects of Substance Abuse, Health, and Mental Health*, DOI 10.1007/978-0-387-78303-1_1, © Springer Science+Business Media New York 2014

and health behaviors, and mental health problems in the active military and their impact on the productivity and readiness of the active duty armed forces across the world. Findings are based on the analyses of the 10 comprehensive Department of Defense Surveys of Health Related Behaviors Among Active Duty Military Personnel (HRB surveys) conducted from 1980 to 2008 (see Bray et al., 2009, 2010).

Productivity is viewed here not in terms of the production of goods but in terms of workforce productivity and the readiness of military personnel to perform their military mission. Throughout the book's discussion of military productivity and readiness, attention is given to the role of deployment and combat experience. Our focus centers on the active duty military force, although for the OIF/OEF conflicts the Reserve components have been called upon and played a key role in supporting the military mission at home and abroad. Behavioral health and readiness issues for the Reserve component (which include the Army Reserve, Army National Guard, Navy Reserve, Marine Corps Reserve, Air Force Reserve, and Air National Guard) are examined in Hourani et al. (2012).

1.2   Military Context

U.S. military forces are charged with maintaining national security and supporting peacetime operations. The importance of this military mission has deepened as the number of threats to national security has increased since September 11, 2001, and the military has been increasingly called upon to defend U.S. national interests across the world. The wars in Iraq and Afghanistan have been particularly demanding and present many challenges for military leaders, service members, and their families. Repeated deployments pose social, economic, mental, and physical challenges. Lengthy separations and combat exposure often lead to worry and anxiety, to psychological health problems as service members return from deployments, to relationship difficulties related to reintegration, and to needed adjustments for physical and psychological wounds (Joint Mental Health Advisory Team 7, 2011; MacDermid Wadsworth & Riggs, 2011; U.S. Department of the Army, 2012).

Indeed, the pressures and stresses associated with military service and deployment in unfamiliar and often dangerous environments may result in and be exacerbated by substance abuse, poor physical health or health-related challenges, and preexisting or recently developed mental health problems. These problems in turn affect the productivity of military personnel and the physical and mental readiness of the force to perform its mission.

Readiness or fitness of the force has traditionally focused on physical fitness and encompassed such components as strength, endurance, flexibility, and mobility (Roy, Springer, McNulty, & Butler, 2010). More recently, due in large measure to the unprecedented demands from the sustained conflicts in Iraq and Afghanistan, the concept of fitness has been broadening to recognize and encompasses the complexity of human behavior. The thrust has been toward a broader, more holistic concept of fitness referred to as Total Force Fitness. Total Force Fitness is an outgrowth of efforts begun by the Army under the direction of General George Casey in 2008 to develop a Comprehensive Soldier Fitness (CSF) program that emphasized physical, emotional, social, family, and spiritual components (Casey, 2011). The new Total Force Fitness paradigm, which was embraced by Admiral Michael Mullen, former Chairman of the Joint Chiefs of Staff (Mullen, 2010), recognizes dimensions of both mind and body, expands on the Army's CSF program, and posits eight fitness domains: behavioral, social, physical, environmental, medical, spiritual, nutritional, and psychological (Jonas et al., 2010). This broader conceptualization of total force fitness builds on current DoD guidance and if fully implemented will contribute to improved productivity of military personnel. More work is needed, however, to clarify the definitions of the fitness components within the eight domains, the metrics for measuring achievement within and across domains, and the training requirements that will be needed for each of these fitness domains.

Although we are not able to consider the integration of all of these domains, the analyses in this book begin to address the overlap in physical, behavioral, and psychological aspects of fitness and their relationship to productivity. Without question, an effective force depends on having healthy and well-trained personnel with a high level of technical competence who are prepared for action. A healthy force is critical to military readiness, and considerable emphasis continues to focus on ways to maintain or improve the health readiness of military personnel (Department of Defense [DoD], 2007; U.S. Department of the Army, 2012).

Resiliency or mental readiness in the face of combat and the psychological stresses of military operations is also essential to the effectiveness of the military force (Thompson & McCreary, 2006). A review of epidemiological studies of troops returning from deployment to Afghanistan and Iraq found that the rates of posttraumatic stress disorder (PTSD) were between 5 and 15 %, and the rates of depression were between 2 and 10 % (Ramchaud, Karney, Osilla, Burns, & Calderone, 2008). More recent population data indicate that the overall PTSD rates across all active duty personnel increased from about 7 % in 2005 to around 11 % in 2008 and that the depression rates were relatively stable during this time (22 % in 2005, 21 % in 2008) (Bray et al., 2010). The physical and mental readiness of each individual service member becomes increasingly important as plans for reset and reductions in the size of the military force proceed (Department of Defense, 2012a; U.S. Department of the Army, 2012).

Substance abuse, poor health, and mental health problems are detrimental to the military in terms of lowered productivity and readiness or fitness and they are also costly to the nation as a whole. A number of studies have examined the enormous economic costs of these often preventable health problems. Despite differences in methodology, these studies have looked at these problems in terms of decreased productivity, absenteeism, increased health care costs, and the costs of criminal justice involvement. For example, cigarette smoking and exposure to tobacco smoke resulted in premature deaths and productivity loss, annually accounting for $96.8 billion (Centers for Disease Control and Prevention, 2008). In 2002, the economic cost of drug abuse to the nation was estimated to be $180.9 billion in terms of health and criminal justice consequences and loss of productivity related to disability, death, and withdrawal from the workforce (Office of National Drug Control Policy, 2004). Excessive alcohol use was estimated to cost $223.5 billion in 2006 in terms of lost productivity, health care costs, criminal justice costs, and other costs (Bouchery, Harwood, Sacks, Simon, & Brewer, 2011).

Substance abuse has economic impacts similar to some other health problems, which together cost the nation trillions of dollars each year. Annually, seven chronic diseases (cancer, diabetes, hypertension, stroke, heart disease, pulmonary conditions, and mental disorders) cost $1.1 trillion in lost productivity and another $277 billion for treatment (DeVol, Bedroussian, Charuworn, & Chatterjee, 2007). The cost of obesity alone is estimated to be $147 billion annually in terms of increased medical spending (Finkelstein, Trogdon, Cohen, & Dietz, 2009). Serious mental illness was estimated to cost $193.2 billion in 2002 in terms of reduced earnings among mentally ill persons (Kessler et al., 2008). Further, cancer accounts for $265 billion, diabetes for $174 billion, and cardiovascular diseases for $291 million each year (Harwood, 2011). The most costly medical conditions in terms of expenditures for health care services nationwide—heart disease, trauma-related disorders, mental disorders, and cancer—all have important components related to potentially intervenable human behavior (http://www.nimh. nih.gov/statistics/4TOT_MC9606.shtml).

In the armed forces, annual tobacco-related costs to the military health system were estimated at $564 million (IOM, 2009). Excessive alcohol use cost DoD an estimated $745 million in reduced readiness and judicial expenses (e.g., prosecution of misconduct charges) (Harwood, Zhang, Dall, Olaiya, & Fagan, 2009). One study calculated the productivity loss resulting from alcohol and illicit substance abuse as being between $411 million and $446 million per year for DoD active service branches. This was estimated as $24 million to $59 million in lost work time, plus an additional $387 million in training and relocation costs to replace personnel who were discharged from service due to alcohol and drug abuse problems (Mehay & Webb, 2007; Friedman, n.d.). In the military, estimates from 2003 of health-related lost productive time translated to roughly 2.5 million lost productive hours per week or an estimated $2 billion per year. When adjusted for inflation, this translates to $2.5 billion in 2012 (Stewart, Ricci, Chee, & Morganstein, 2003; Friedman, n.d.).

1.3   The Active Duty Military Force Across the World

As of September 2011, there were 1.4 million active duty military personnel in the Army, Navy, Marine Corps, and Air Force. Military personnel are stationed on bases and afloat in locations across the world. In 2011, of the total of 1.4 million active duty military personnel, the vast majority—about 1.2 million—were stationed in the United States and its territories. About 81,000 were stationed in Europe and 56,000 were stationed in East Asia and the Pacific. Among Reserve and National Guard personnel, 92,000 personnel were stationed in Iraq as part of

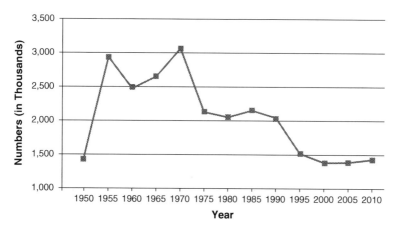

Fig. 1.1 Trends in active duty military personnel, 1950–2010
Source: U.S. Census Bureau, Statistical Abstract 2004–2005 and 2012

OIF and 109,000 were stationed in Afghanistan as part of OEF in 2011 (Department of Defense, 2011a).

The size of the active duty military force has changed over the past decades in response to changing requirements of military operations. As shown in Fig. 1.1, in 1950, the military force was 1.5 million in the period following World War II and increased to about 3.0 million during the early 1950s in response to the Korean War. The force decreased to 2.5 million during the late 1950s and early 1960s but again increased during the late 1960s in response to the Vietnam War. Throughout the 1970s and 1980s, military personnel numbered about 2 million, dropping below that number during the 1990s. The Gulf War in 1991 occurred during this downsizing, while the military force during the conflicts in Iraq and Afghanistan showed small increases. These numbers have since been augmented with members of the Reserve component.

The armed forces have relied on volunteer service since 1973 when President Richard Nixon created the all-volunteer force in response to public dissatisfaction with the draft. This resulted in the smaller, all-volunteer professional military we continue to have today. Over the past 15 years, the active duty military force has averaged about 1.4 million, of whom, in 2011, 565,000 (40 %) were in the Army, 325,000 (23 %) were in the Navy, 201,000 (14 %) were in the Marine Corps, and 333,000 (23 %) were in the Air Force. Of the 1.4 million active duty members, about 1.2 million are enlisted personnel.

The active duty force is composed predominantly of young men. In 2009, nearly half (45 %) of the active duty military personnel were aged 25 or younger. The proportion of women has increased over the past several decades. In 1950, military women numbered about 22,000 or 1.5 % of the force. The number increased slowly during the 1950s and 1960s and more rapidly during the 1970s. By 1980, the 171,000 active duty women constituted 8 % of the force. Since the 1980s, military women have numbered about 200,000 and now constitute about 14 % of the force.

The enlisted force is 72 % white, 17 % African American, and 11 % Hispanic. About 80 % of the active duty force has less than a bachelor's degree; 96 % of the officers have a bachelor's degree or higher compared with about 5 % of the enlisted personnel. A little over half (55 %) of the active duty personnel are married. The force is becoming older, more racially diverse, and more highly educated. Of military accessions, 92.9 % now have a high school diploma (Department of Defense, 2011b; Office of the Under Secretary of Defense, 2009). However, in order to meet recruitment targets since OIF/OEF, the Army's percentage of recruits with high school diplomas has dropped from 94 % in 2003 to 70.7 % in 2007, and scores on the armed forces aptitude tests have tumbled significantly (http://www.slate.com/articles/news_and_politics/war_stories/2008/01/dumb_and_dumber.html). Chapter 2 provides additional information about the demographic composition of the active force and how it has changed over the years.

1.4 Influences on Military Productivity and Readiness

The construct of productivity is a continually evolving aspect of work performance in civilian organizations and is even more intricate in the military context. The ability of military personnel to successfully meet the demands placed on them is affected by a number of pressures that influence their level of productivity and readiness to serve. Productivity of the military force is viewed here in terms of the ability to perform this mission through a framework of "performance loss," the extent to which time at work is spent with energy focused on something other than the job. This framework measures the (a) degree of reduced work capacity, (b) time away from task, and (c) prevalence within the organization (Ricci & Chee, 2005).

As noted earlier, several of the issues currently affecting the overall effectiveness of the military force include substance use, overall health status and health behaviors, and mental health problems. Other important considerations are the impact of long and multiple deployments and combat experience, the stresses of managing home life during separations, the increasing numbers of injured personnel, reintegration to society and family life after returning from deployment, and challenges in maintaining a military force of sufficient size to meet current demands. We examine these factors in the following sections.

1.4.1 Substance Abuse

Research in both civilian and military settings shows a clear relationship between substance abuse and productivity loss. Military concerns over substance abuse by military personnel emerged during the 1970s with the recognition of the problem of drug use among troops during the Vietnam War. These concerns intensified following the 1981 crash of a military plane on the flight deck of the aircraft carrier Nimitz.

Autopsies of 14 Navy personnel killed in the crash showed evidence of marijuana use among 6 of the 13 sailors and nonprescription antihistamine use by the pilot. The final conclusion was that the illicit drug use may have been a contributing factor in the accident. In response, DoD initiated its policy of zero tolerance accompanied by mandatory drug testing for all military personnel. Illicit drug use in the past month among the military personnel subsequently decreased from 28 % in 1980 to 2 % from 1992 to 2002, although it has since increased (Bray et al., 2009, 2010), primarily due to increases in prescription drug misuse. Prescription drug misuse, or nonmedical use of these drugs, increased between 2002 and 2008, while rates of illicit drug use excluding prescription drug misuse continued at the low rates observed in 2002 around 2 %. The observed increase in prescription drug misuse was largely driven by high rates of abuse of pain medications (Bray, Rae Olmsted, & Williams, 2012). Of note, misuse of prescription drugs to relieve pain suggests a very different motivation for use than that of getting "high" typically associated with illicit drug use. Nonetheless, it may point to different but equally concerning issues of pain and pain management among these personnel.

The Department of Defense has struggled with issues of productivity loss related to alcohol abuse in terms of reduced readiness and higher force management costs in addition to increased medical costs and judicial expenses incurred because of excessive alcohol use. Concerns over alcohol abuse among military personnel also emerged during the 1970s and have intensified over time with the growing recognition of the significance of the impact of alcohol abuse on military productivity loss. Several studies have documented the impact of excessive alcohol use on productivity loss among military personnel (Fisher, Hoffman, Austin-Lane, & Kao, 2000; Mattiko, Rae Olmsted, Brown, & Bray, 2011; Stahre, Brewer, Fonseca, & Naimi, 2009). For example, Mattiko et al. (2011) found a curvilinear dose–response relationship with productivity loss and drinking levels. Higher levels of drinking were associated with higher rates of alcohol problems, but problem rates were notably higher for heavy drinkers who showed over twice the rate of self-reported productivity loss than moderate/heavy drinkers. To be sure, alcohol abuse in the military is a complex issue that appears related to the military's culture of heavy drinking, reduced prices for alcohol on military installations, use of alcohol to relieve work-related stress, and increased use associated with deployment, deployment liberty, and combat exposure (Ames, Cunradi, Moore, & Stern, 2007; Bray et al., 2009; Bray, Brown, & Williams, 2013; Federman, Bray, & Kroutil, 2000; Jacobson et al., 2008).

1.4.2 Health Status and Health Behaviors

The physical health of military personnel is a vital component of productivity and readiness that affects work performance and absenteeism in the military. Being free from injury and being in good physical condition have long been recognized as critical to readiness and productivity. The 2008 Physical Activity Guidelines for Americans (Department of Health and Human Services, 2008) makes an important distinction between health-related fitness and performance-related fitness that has implications for the military. Health-related fitness emphasizes the levels of exercise and physical training that are needed to promote and improve cardiovascular and muscular fitness and reduce the risk of disease or injury. This type of fitness is encouraged for all Americans. Performance-related fitness focuses on the levels and amount of physical training needed to achieve a particular goal such as climbing a high peak or completing a distance run within a specified time limit. The military needs both types of fitness but gives high emphasis to performance fitness because it is related to mission accomplishment (Roy et al., 2010) and, of course, to productivity. In this framework, performance fitness varies across individuals and units depending on their military jobs and the related task requirements. Performance requirements will be quite different for soldiers who will be carrying back packs and perhaps other equipment across rough terrain in Afghanistan than it will be for aircraft mechanics.

It should be no surprise that poor physical fitness as well as overweight and obesity are associated with productivity loss and absenteeism among military personnel (Kyrolainen et al., 2008). Similarly, physical illness and injury limit the ability of personnel to perform at peak levels and have been shown to be related to missed work among both active duty and Reserve component personnel (Bray et al., 2009; Hourani et al., 2007). Further, the impact of health on military productivity may be exacerbated by combat experience largely because of higher risks of illness or injury in adverse environments. Consistent with this logic, Helmer et al. (2007) found that veterans returning from Iraq and Afghanistan reported a number of physical health concerns and exposures to poor health conditions and toxins.

1.4.3 Mental Health Problems

Occupational and family stressors and mental health problems affect active duty military personnel's overall job performance and productivity, and mental health problems can emerge from military service. Hourani, Williams, and Kress (2006) found that the military personnel with high rates of work and family stress had higher rates of mental health problems and productivity loss than those with lower stress. War exposure in Iraq, Afghanistan, and other locations resulted in PTSD symptoms among service members and overall poorer health and functioning (Vinokur, Pierce, Lewandowski-Romps, Hobfoll, & Galea, 2011). Combat duty in Iraq was associated with high rates of utilization of mental health services and attrition from military service after deployment (Hoge, Auchterlonie, & Milliken, 2006). Skyrocketing suicide rates not only affect family and friends but also take a serious toll on both unit members and military caregivers (Carr, 2011). From the beginning of the wars in Iraq and Afghanistan through 2011, well over 211,000 combat veterans have been treated by the Veterans Administration for PTSD, and another estimated 200,000 with PTSD symptoms have sought care elsewhere or not at all (*USA Today*, 2011).

1.4.4 Deployment and Combat Experience

Among the most pressing issues for the military are the challenges stemming from long and repeated deployments. Approximately, 1 million military personnel served in Iraq between 2003 and 2011, and more than 2.3 million personnel have been deployed to Iraq, Afghanistan, or both. More than half (58 %) of the personnel who have served in Iraq or Afghanistan have been deployed more than once (Martinez & Bingham, 2011). Many service members deployed to Iraq and Afghanistan have been placed in high-risk situations that are highly stressful. One study found that 25 % of returning veterans had a mental health diagnosis, and more than half of these had more than one such diagnosis. Personnel most at risk for a mental health diagnosis were 18–24-year-olds and those with the most combat exposure (Seal, Bertenthal, Miner, Sen, & Marmar, 2007). Explosions, motor vehicle crashes, transport, and falls place OIF/OEF veterans at risk for traumatic brain injury (TBI), which is highly comorbid with PTSD (Schneiderman, Braver, & Kang, 2008). Pre- and post-deployment health assessments indicated decreases in self-ratings of health and increases in behavioral health referrals following deployment (Medical Surveillance Monthly Report, 2007). However, findings from the Millennium Cohort Study found that deployment was not associated with decreased physical health status (Smith et al., 2007). The relationship between behavioral effects of combat exposure is a complex one as evidenced by a study, showing that PTSD mediates the relationship between mild TBI and a number of health and psychosocial functioning indices in OIF/OEF veterans (Pietrzak, Johnson, Goldstein, Malley, & Southwick, 2009).

1.4.5 Stress During Separations

A great deal of emphasis has recently been placed on stress and challenges experienced by families who remain at home during deployments (Mansfield et al., 2010). Indeed, separations due to military exercises, school attendance, or deployment can have substantial negative effects on the psychological and physical well-being of military family members, even more so than other aspects of military life such as the risk of injury or death, relocations, or foreign residence (Burrell, Adams, Durand, & Castro, 2006).

Of equal concern is the stress due to family separation experienced by service members when they are deployed. With the increased presence of technology-assisted communications, service members have unprecedented contact, sometimes on a daily basis, with their families. Although increased communication may help service members feel closer to their families, it also can be frustrating to be aware of daily hassles without the ability to more fully address them. Research shows that having a spouse present serves as a stabilizing force for military members. For example, Bray, Spira, and Lane (2011) found that single service members and married service members who had deployed without their spouses had higher rates of mental health problems and behavioral problems compared to their counterparts who were married and whose spouses were present.

1.4.6 Injury

Injuries among personnel have long been a concern for the military because they are costly and represent a complex problem that impacts the military's strength and ability to respond to its mission. This concern has increased with the higher injury rates that have resulted from regular and frequent combat deployments in support of OIF/OEF. As of April 2012, almost 32,000 military personnel had been wounded in action in Iraq and almost 16,000 had been wounded in Afghanistan (Department of Defense, 2012b). However, the high rates of injury among combat-deployed personnel were not solely the result of direct combat. Of the 13,000 military casualties examined during OIF, about a quarter were wounded in action, while the remainder were the result of disease and non-combat injuries (Zouris, Wade, & Magno, 2008).

As we discuss in Chap. 4, injuries have been identified as the single most significant medical impediment to military readiness and hence to productivity and the largest health problem faced by the military (Jones, Canham-Chervak, & Sleet, 2010). As an outgrowth of recent efforts to address the injury problem, the current military environment places high importance on injury prevention and control.

1.4.7 Problems in Reintegration

Another area that has received increasing attention is the tremendous strain of readjustment to returning to civilian life following combat deployment. In prior conflicts, service members were deployed to forward combat areas, returning to relatively safe rear bases to restock, receive new instructions, and rest and recuperate. Following their combat deployment, service members took a long trip home, followed by demobilization at their home base. This allowed for a gradual decompression. By contrast, today's missions require continual vigilance, whether on convoy, patrolling the streets of an Iraqi village or the hills of Afghanistan, or returning to base camp. In addition, service members can be in a firefight one day, and a week later can be home with their families. The skill set required to be a successful service member can help individuals throughout their subsequent civilian life. However, it is impractical to expect service members to simply "turn off" the vigilance and aggressiveness that helps them survive and accomplish a mission in-country once they return to their families back home.

Such transitions can take months, and some personnel will require assistance beyond existing programs and efforts that have currently been implemented (IOM, 2013). One progressive approach by the National Guard includes pre-deployment preparation retreats geared toward preparing service members, and often family members, on what to expect during deployment as well as post-deployment reintegration retreats focused on facilitating the transition back to home life. Although laudable, there is unfortunately little research as to the impact such programs have on reducing substance abuse and mental health problems among service members or their families.

1.4.8 Job Satisfaction and Retention

Both effective recruitment and effective retention are essential to maintain a strong fighting force. During periods when traditional recruiting efforts have not been adequate to reach recruitment targets, the military has sometimes had to lower standards for admission. Issues such as minimum scores on the Armed Forces Qualifying Test (AFQT) and subsequent determination of military occupational specialty based upon Armed Services Vocational Aptitude Battery (ASVAB) scores that allow recruits to opt out of stressful experiences during basic training, and a lowered threshold for passing special operations trainings, have all been reconsidered during the years when recruitment and retention is low. Therefore, the quality and skills of personnel admitted into the services and specific jobs is related to individual and family stress. Job satisfaction can also be important to job performance; this relationship is likely affected by personality traits, job autonomy, and job complexity (Judge, Thoresen, Bono, & Patton, 2001).

1.5 Programmatic Responses to Military Productivity and Readiness

As we show throughout this book, substance abuse, poor health practices, and mental health problems as well as the impact of military conditions and deployment all detract from the productivity and readiness of the active duty military force. Abuse of alcohol and illicit drugs can impair work performance or pose a danger to others if personnel are under the influence of alcohol or drugs, or recovering from their effects, when carrying out military duties. Use of alcohol and other drugs can also create personnel or family problems that can interfere with job performance. In the military any use of illicit drugs is considered abuse because it is against military policy and detracts from military discipline.

To address these issues, DoD has put in place regulations, policies, programs, and campaigns to encourage and support healthy lifestyles, to deter and prevent problem behaviors, and to treat substance abuse issues, physical health problems, and mental health problems that arise. Much of the healthy lifestyle emphasis for the active force has been consolidated under the broad umbrella of health promotion, beginning in the mid-1980s. Indeed, health promotion in the military emerged as an outgrowth of drug and alcohol abuse problems that surfaced in the 1970s among troops during the Vietnam War and growing recognition of the significance of the problem. Beginning in 1972, the military began a series of policy directives, which were further elaborated on throughout the 1970s and 1980s. A formal, coordinated health promotion policy was instituted in 1986, integrating programs in six broad areas: smoking prevention and cessation, physical fitness, nutrition, stress management, alcohol and other drug abuse prevention, and hypertension prevention. These policies have guided military programs over the past 25 years.

The emphasis on health promotion in the active force was further reinforced with the publication of *Healthy People 2000* (Public Health Service, 1991). Among other things, the report focused additional attention in the military on the need for prevention and reduction of unhealthy substance abuse behaviors such as heavy drinking, cigarette smoking, and illicit drug abuse. It also encouraged the improvement of physical health through exercise and proper diet and the prevention and treatment of illnesses and injuries. In 2000, the publication of *Healthy People 2010* updated and expanded the earlier set of objectives (Department of Health and Human Services, 2000). Most recently, *Healthy People 2020* was launched in 2010 with a revised 10-year agenda for further improving the nation's health (Department of Health and Human Services, 2012). The active duty military has been proactive in establishing or adopting a variety of substance abuse and health-related programs intended to encourage and motivate service members to reduce negative substance use behaviors and to increase or engage in positive health behaviors. These programs and their goals are described in Chap. 7. Unfortunately, despite these efforts, there are still substantial substance abuse issues and problems among service members that need attention. A recent IOM report identified a high rate of substance use disorders among active duty service members and veterans (IOM, 2012) and indicated a need for a culture change in the military to realize further progress in reducing substance use and called for more effective approaches for addressing substance use disorders.

In addition, the stresses and challenges of combat exposure combined with recurring and extended deployments during OIF/OEF have focused considerable attention on mental health issues among military personnel. To address these concerns the military has commissioned a large number of studies and developed and expanded a variety of programs that target prevention, intervention, and treatment of mental health problems. These efforts, which are described more fully in Chap. 7 of this book, have been directed toward problems and issues of stress management, combat and operational stress control, depression, anxiety, PTSD, mild TBI, suicide prevention, and resiliency training.

1.6 Overview of This Book

This book examines the predictors and correlates of substance abuse, health status and health behaviors, and mental health problems and the impact of these factors on the productivity and readiness of the active duty military force across the world. We also consider the effects on military productivity and readiness of factors such as deployment and combat exposures, illness and injury, and other military experiences.

Data are drawn from a series of 10 HRB surveys spanning a 28-year period from 1980 to 2008 (see Bray et al., 2009). Analyses focus on these behaviors and issues for the aggregate DoD active duty force, rather than separately for the four individual DoD services (Army, Navy, Marine Corps, Air Force) and concentrate on findings from the 2008 HRB survey. Selected analyses for the four active duty services are discussed in the text as appropriate.

1.6.1   Conceptual Framework

Analyses are organized and guided by our conceptual framework that considers substance abuse, health status and health behaviors, and mental health problems as important determinants of military productivity and readiness. In our framework, substance abuse, health, and mental health are viewed as intermediate outcomes, and productivity and readiness are viewed as final outcomes. These intermediate and final outcomes are influenced by background characteristics that include sociodemographic characteristics, psychosocial characteristics, and military conditions. Sociodemographic characteristics examined here include age, gender, race/ethnicity, education, family status, and the presence of children in the home. Psychosocial characteristics include risk-taking perspectives, spirituality, a history of physical or sexual abuse, and mechanisms for coping with stress. Military conditions include pay grade, branch of service, deployment and combat experience, and military location (within or outside the continental United States). This framework is illustrated in Fig. 1.2.

Chapter 2 describes how we measured each of the types of variables in Fig. 1.2. Using these measures, we conducted analyses of the predictors and correlates of substance abuse, health behaviors and health conditions, and mental health problems.

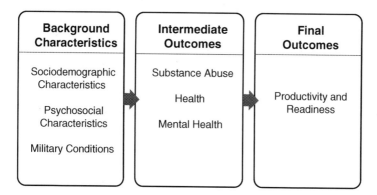

Fig. 1.2 Conceptual framework guiding analyses

We then examined the role of these intermediate outcomes on productivity and readiness of the active duty military force. These analyses are presented in subsequent chapters.

1.6.2 The Health-Related Behavior Surveys

The analyses presented in this book are based on data from the 1980 to 2008 Department of Defense Surveys of Health Related Behaviors Among Active Duty Military Personnel. The first of these comprehensive worldwide surveys was conducted in 1980 under the direction of the Office of the Assistant Secretary of Defense for Health Affairs. The initial survey was primarily focused on substance abuse issues. Subsequent surveys, also conducted under the direction of the Office of the Assistant Secretary of Defense for Health Affairs, continued this theme but were broadened to include other constructs. All of the surveys have been used as a broad barometer of how health and substance abuse programs (and mental health programs since the terrorist attacks of September 11, 2001) have been working and as a signal of where adjustments in programs and policies may be needed. Eleven HRB surveys have now been conducted for the active military—in 1980, 1982, 1985, 1988, 1992, 1995, 1998, 2002, 2005, 2008, and 2011. The first survey was conducted by Burt Associates, Incorporated, of Bethesda, Maryland (Burt, Biegel, Carnes, & Farley, 1980) and the 1982–2008 surveys were conducted by RTI International of Research Triangle Park, North Carolina (Bray et al., 1983, 1986, 1988, 1992, 1995, 1999, 2003, 2006, 2009). The 2011 survey was conducted by ICF International, but only an overview of results have been released at the time of this writing (Barlas, Higgins, Pflieger, & Diecker, 2013). The 2011 survey was not included in the analyses of this book because extensive changes in the methodology (both mode of data collection and questionnaire items) preclude direct comparison with the 1980–2008 iterations of the survey.

The content and methodology of the 1980–2008 surveys have been very similar over the years to enable monitoring of trends in substance abuse, health behaviors, and mental health problems among military personnel. However, some content changes have been introduced across the surveys to reflect newly emerging issues and concerns. For example, beginning in 1985, the surveys included a broadened focus on health behaviors and health promotion, and the 1995 survey included additional questions on *Healthy People* objectives. The 2002 survey included additional questions on mental health services, barriers to receiving health services, men's health issues, oral health, and problem gambling. In 2005, revisions were made to the alcohol use items to incorporate the Alcohol Use Disorders Identification Test (AUDIT). Questions were also added to assess nicotine dependence; questions on illicit drug use were revised to add descriptions of drug use categories, and questions on sexual enhancers were added. Questions were also added to better assess nutrition and overweight, use of complementary or alternative medicine treatments, mental health problems (depression, serious psychological distress, generalized anxiety disorder, PTSD), and deployment and its effects. In 2008, further revisions to the illicit drug use items were made (such that questions about illegal drugs and prescription drugs were asked separately, and questions about "analgesics" were changed to "pain relievers" to reduce ambiguity for respondents) to enable more detailed consideration of the use of illegal drugs and nonmedical use of prescription drugs. In addition, improved measures of deployment were added along with new measures to examine combat exposure and to screen for the presence of possible mild TBI.

1.6.3 Overview of Chapters

The findings of this book are presented in seven chapters. Chapter 2 describes the methodology for conducting the 1980–2008 HRB surveys, including the sampling design, instrumentation, data collection, survey performance rates, key definitions and measures, and analytical approach. It also presents information on the sociodemographic composition of the active duty military and briefly examines the validity of self-report data for the measures that were included in the surveys. Chapters 3–5 consider the prevalence and correlates of key intermediate outcomes: substance abuse (Chap. 3), health behaviors and health status (Chap. 4), and stress and mental health problems (Chap. 5). Each of these three chapters examines trends in the prevalence of key indicators and the sociodemographic, psychosocial, and military predictors of those measures. Where possible, comparisons are made regarding the prevalence of key indicators of the health and behavioral health of the military population to the civilian population. The HRB survey series is the source of data for most of the tables and figures included in the report.

Chapter 6 presents trends in productivity loss associated with substance abuse health behaviors and health status and mental health problems as well as the correlates and predictors of productivity loss. It then presents and examines a health and behavioral health model of productivity loss that integrates the key concepts and measures of substance abuse, physical health, and mental health considered in Chaps. 3–5 with an emphasis on how they relate and converge to impact productivity among active duty personnel. The model provides a comprehensive assessment of how health and behavioral health factors, taken together, affect productivity in the military.

Chapter 7 provides a review of key findings and their implications regarding the predictors of substance abuse, physical health problems, and mental health problems and their effects on workforce productivity and readiness of military personnel. It also considers study limitations and examines the programmatic approaches of the military to address challenges of servicemen along with significant issues requiring further research.

It is our hope that these findings will provide new information and insights about how health and behavioral health contribute to improved quality of life of service members and their families and in turn the quality of the military.

References

Adler, A. B., Bliese, P. D., & Castro, C. A. (Eds.). (2011). *Deployment psychology*. Washington, DC: American Psychological Association.

Ames, G. M., Cunradi, C. B., Moore, R. S., & Stern, P. (2007). Military culture and drinking behavior among U.S. Navy careerists. *Journal of Studies on Alcohol and Drugs, 68*(3), 336–344.

Barlas, F.M., Higgins, W.B., Pflieger, J.S., & Diecker, K. (2013). *2011 Department of Defense Health Related Behaviors Survey of Active Duty Military Personnel: Executive Summary*. Retrieved from http://tricare.mil/tma/dhcape/surveys/coresurveys/surveyhealthrelatedbehaviors/downloads/Final%202011%20HRB%20Active%20Duty%20Survey%20Exec%20Summary.pdf

Bouchery, E. E., Harwood, H. J., Sacks, J. J., Simon, C. J., & Brewer, R. D. (2011). Economic costs of excessive alcohol consumption in the U.S., 2006. *American Journal of Preventive Medicine, 41*(5), 516–524.

Bray, R. M., Brown, J. M., & Williams, J. (2013). Trends in binge and heavy drinking and alcohol consumption-related problems: Implications of combat exposure in the U.S. Military. *Substance Use and Misuse, 48*(10), 799–810. doi:10.3109/10826084.2013.796990.

Bray, R. M., Guess, L. L., Mason, R. E., Hubbard, R. L., Smith, D. G., Marsden, M. E., et al. (1983). *1982 worldwide survey of alcohol and Non-medical drug use among military personnel (RTI/2317/01-01F)*. Research Triangle Park, NC: Research Triangle Institute.

Bray, R. M., Hourani, L. L., Rae Olmsted, K. L., Witt, M., Brown, J. M., Pemberton, M. R., et al. (2006). *2005 Department of Defense survey of health related behaviors among active duty military personnel (RTI/7841/106-FR)*. Research Triangle Park, NC: Research Triangle Institute.

Bray, R. M., Hourani, L. L., Rae, K. L., Dever, J. A., Brown, J. M., Vincus, A. A., et al. (2003). *2002 Department of Defense survey of health related behaviors among military personnel: Final report* (prepared for the Assistant Secretary of Defense [Health Affairs], U.S. Department of Defense, Cooperative Agreement No. DAMD17-00-2-0057/RTI/7841/006-FR). Research Triangle Park, NC: Research Triangle Institute.

Bray, R. M., Kroutil, L. A., Luckey, J. W., Wheeless, S. C., Iannacchione, V. G., Anderson, D. W., et al. (1992). *1992 Worldwide survey of substance abuse and health behaviors among military personnel*. Research Triangle Park, NC: Research Triangle Institute.

Bray, R. M., Kroutil, L. A., Wheeless, S. C., Marsden, M. E., Bailey, S. L., Fairbank, J. A., et al. (1995). *1995 Department of Defense survey of health related behaviors among military personnel (DoD Contract No. DASO1-94-C-0140)*. Research Triangle Park, NC: Research Triangle Institute.

Bray, R. M., Marsden, M. E., Guess, L. L., Wheeless, S. C., Iannacchione, V. G., & Keesling, S. R. (1988). *1988 worldwide survey of substance abuse and health behaviors among military personnel*. Research Triangle Park, NC: Research Triangle Institute.

Bray, R. M., Marsden, M. E., Guess, L. L., Wheeless, S. C., Pate, D. K., Dunteman, G. H., et al. (1986). *1985 Worldwide survey of alcohol and nonmedical drug use among military personnel*. Research Triangle Park, NC: Research Triangle Institute.

Bray, R. M., Pemberton, M. R., Hourani, L. L., Witt, M., Rae Olmsted, K. L., Brown, J. M., et al. (2009). *2008 Department of Defense survey of health related behaviors among active duty military personnel*. Report prepared for TRICARE Management Activity, Office of the Assistant Secretary of Defense (Health Affairs) and U.S. Coast Guard. Research Triangle Park, NC: Research Triangle Institute.

Bray, R. M., Pemberton, M., Lane, M. E., Hourani, L. L., Mattiko, M., & Babeu, L. A. (2010). Substance use and mental health trends among U.S. military active duty personnel: Key findings from the 2008 DoD Health Behavior Survey. *Military Medicine, 175*(6), 390–399.

Bray, R. M., Rae Olmsted, K. L., & Williams, J. (2012). Misuse of prescription pain medications in U.S. active duty service members. In: B. K. Wiederhold (Ed.), *Pain syndromes: From recruitment to returning troops: Vol. 91. NATO Science for Peace and Security Series E: Human and Societal Dynamics* (pp. 3–16). Amsterdam, Netherlands: IOS Press.

Bray, R. M., Sanchez, R. P., Ornstein, M. L., Lentine, D., Vincus, A. A., et al. (1999). *1998 Department of Defense survey of health related behaviors among military personnel*: Final report (prepared for the Assistant Secretary of Defense [Health Affairs], U.S. Department of Defense, Cooperative Agreement No. DAMD17-96-2-6021, RTI/7034/006-FR). Research Triangle Park, NC: Research Triangle Institute.

Bray, R. M., Spira, J. L., & Lane, M. E. (2011). The single service member: Substance use, stress and mental health issues. In S. MacDermid Wadsworth & D. Riggs (Eds.), *Risk and resilience in U.S. military families*. New York: Springer.

Burrell, L. M., Adams, G. A., Durand, D. B., & Castro, C. A. (2006). The impact of military lifestyle demands on well-being, Army, and family outcomes. *Armed Forces and Society, 33*(1), 43–58.

Burt, M. A., Biegel, M. M., Carnes, Y., & Farley, E. C. (1980). *Worldwide survey of non-medical drug use and alcohol use among military personnel: 1980*. Bethesda, MD: Burt Associates.

Carr, R. B. (2011). When a soldier commits suicide in Iraq: Impact on unit and caregivers. *Psychiatry, 74*(2), 95–106.

Casey, G. W., Jr. (2011). Comprehensive soldier fitness: A vision for psychological resilience in the U.S. Army. *American Psychologist, 66*, 1–3.

Centers for Disease Control and Prevention. (2008). *Morbidity and Mortality Weekly, 57*(45), 1226–1228.

Department of Defense. (2007). *Task force on the future of military care*. Final Report. A Subcommittee of the Defense Health Board.

Department of Defense. (2011a). *Active duty military personnel strengths by regional area and by country*. Retrieved September 30, 2011, from http://siadapp.dmdc.mil/personnel/MILITARY/history/hst1109.pdf

Department of Defense. (2011b). *Demographics 2010. Profile of the Military Community*. Arlington, VA: DoD.

Department of Defense. (2012a). *Defense budget priorities and choices*. www.defense.gov/news/Defense_Budget_Priorities.pdf

Department of Defense. (2012b). *U.S. casualty status*. Retrieved April 18, 2012, from www.defense.gov

Department of Health and Human Services. (2000). *Healthy people 2010: Understanding and improving health* (2nd ed.). Washington, DC: U.S. Government Printing Office.

Department of Health and Human Services. (2008). *2008 physical activity guidelines for Americans*. Washington, DC: DHHS.

Department of Health and Human Services. (2012). Office of Disease Prevention and Health Promotion. *Healthy People 2020*. Washington, DC. Retrieved January 25, 2013, from http://healthypeople.gov/2020/topicsobjectives2020/overview.aspx?topicid=40

DeVol, R., Bedroussian, A., Charuworn, A., & Chatterjee, A. (2007). *An unhealthy America: The economic burden of chronic disease—Charting a new course to save lives and increase productivity and economic growth*. Santa Monica, CA: Milkin Institute.

Federman, B., Bray, R. M., & Kroutil, L. A. (2000). Relationships between substance use and recent deployments among women and men in the military. *Military Psychology, 12*(3), 205–220.

Finkelstein, E. A., Trogdon, J. G., Cohen, J. W., & Dietz, W. (2009). Annual medical spending attributable to obesity: Payer and service-specific estimates. *Health Affairs, 28*(5), w822–w831.

Fisher, C. A., Hoffman, K. J., Austin-Lane, J., & Kao, T. C. (2000). The relationship between heavy alcohol use and work productivity loss in active duty military personnel: A secondary analysis of the 1995 Department of Defense Worldwide Survey. *Military Medicine, 165*(5), 355–361.

Friedman, S. M. (n.d.). The inflation calculator. Retrieved June 4, 2013, from http://www.westegg.com/inflation/

Harwood, H. (2011). *Recent findings on the economic impacts of substance abuse*. Presented to the American Psychological Association 2011 Science Leadership Conference, Psychological Science and Substance Abuse.

Harwood, H. J., Zhang, Y., Dall, T. M., Olaiya, S. T., & Fagan, N. K. (2009). Economic implications of reduced binge drinking among the military health system's TRICARE prime plan beneficiaries. *Military Medicine, 174*(7), 728–736.

Helmer, D. A., Rissignol, M., Blatt, M., Agarwal, R., Teichman, R., & Lange, G. (2007). Health and exposure concerns of veterans deployed to Iraq and Afghanistan. *Journal of Occupational and Environmental Medicine, 49*(5), 475–480.

Hoge, C. W., Auchterlonie, J. L., & Milliken, C. S. (2006). Mental health problems, use of mental health services, and attrition from military service after returning from deployment to Iraq or Afghanistan. *Journal of the American Medical Association, 295*(9), 1023–1032.

Hourani, L. L., Bray, R. M., Marsden, M. E., Witt, M., Vandermaas-Peeler, R, Schleffler, S., et al. (2007). *2006 Department of Defense survey of health related behaviors in the Reserve Component.* Report prepared for the U.S. Department of Defense (Cooperative Agreement No. DAMD17-00-2-0057).

Hourani, L. L., Lane, M. E., Scheffler, S. A., Williams, J., Peeler, J. R., Aspinwall, K. R., et al. (2012). *Department of Defense health related behaviors reserve component survey* (Report No. RTI/1586/004/FR). Prepared for Department of Defense.

Hourani, L. L., Williams, T. V., & Kress, A. M. (2006). Stress, mental health, and job performance among active duty military personnel: Findings from the 2002 Department of Defense Health related Behaviors Survey. *Military Medicine, 171*(9), 849–846.

Institute of Medicine (IOM). (2009). *Combating tobacco use in military and veteran populations.* Washington, DC: The National Academies Press.

Institute of Medicine (IOM). (2012). *Substance use disorders in the U.S. armed forces.* Washington, DC: The National Academies Press.

Institute of Medicine (IOM). (2013). *Assessment of readjustment needs of veterans, service members, and their families.* Washington, DC: The National Academies Press.

Jacobson, I. G., Ryan, M. A. K., Hooper, T. I., Smith, T. C., Amoroso, P. J., Boyko, E. J., et al. (2008). Alcohol use and alcohol-related problems before and after military combat deployment. *Journal of the American Medical Association, 300*(6), 663–675.

Joint Mental Health Advisory Team 7 (2011). *Operation Enduring Freedom 2010, Afghanistan.* Office of the Surgeon General, U.S. Army and Office of the command Surgeon, Headquarters, U.S. Central Command, and Office of the Command Surgeon, U.S. Forces Afghanistan.

Jonas, W. B., O'Connor, F. G., Deuster, P., Peck, J., Shake, C., & Frost, S. S. (2010). Why total force fitness? *Military Medicine, 175*(8), 6–13.

Jones, B. H., Canham-Chervak, M., & Sleet, D. A. (2010). An evidence-based public health approach to injury priorities and prevention: Recommendations for the U.S. Military. *American Journal of Preventive Medicine, 38*(1 Suppl), S1–S10.

Judge, T. A., Thoresen, C. J., Bono, J. E., & Patton, G. K. (2001). The job satisfaction-job performance relationship: A qualitative and quantitative review. *Psychological Bulletin, 127*(3), 376–407.

Kessler, R. C., Heeringa, S., Lakoma, M. D., Petukhova, M., Rupp, A. E., Schoenbaum, M., et al. (2008). Individual and societal effects of mental disorders on earnings in the United States: Results from the National Comorbidity Survey Replication. *American Journal of Psychiatry, 165*, 703–711.

Kyrolainen, H., Hakkinen, K., Kautiainen, H., Santtila, M., Pihlainen, K., & Hakkinen, A. (2008). Physical fitness, BMI and sickness absence in male military personnel. *Occupational Medicine, 58*(4), 251–256.

MacDermid Wadsworth, S., & Riggs, D. (Eds.). (2011). *Risk and resilience in U.S. military families.* New York: Springer.

Mansfield, A. J., Kaufman, J. S., Marshall, S. W., Gaynes, B. N., Morrissey, J. P., & Engel, C. C. (2010). Deployment and use of mental health services among U.S. army wives. *New England Journal of Medicine, 362*, 101–109.

Martinez, L., & Bingham, B. (2011). U.S. Veterans: By the numbers. *ABC News*, November 11.

Mattiko, M., Rae Olmsted, K. L., Brown, J. M., & Bray, R. M. (2011). Alcohol use and negative consequences among active duty military personnel. *Addictive Behaviors, 36*, 608–614.

Mehay, S., & Webb, N. J. (2007). Workplace drug prevention programs: Does zero tolerance work? *Applied Economics, 39*, 2743–2751.

Mullen, M. (2010). On total force fitness in war and peace. *Military Medicine, 175*(8), 1–2.

Office of National Drug Control Policy. (2004). *The economic costs of drug abuse in the United States, 1992–2002*. Washington, DC: Executive Office of the President.

Office of the Under Secretary of Defense. (2009). *Population representation in the military services, fiscal year 2010*. Retrieved May 22, 2012, from http://prhome.defense.gov/rfm/MPP/ACCESSION%20Policy/PopRep2010/

Pietrzak, R. H., Johnson, D. C., Goldstein, M. B., Malley, J. C., & Southwick, S. M. (2009). Posttraumatic stress disorder mediates the relationship between mild traumatic brain injury and health and psychosocial functioning in veterans of Operations Enduring Freedom and Iraqi Freedom. *Journal of Nervous and Mental Disease, 197*, 748–753.

Ramchaud, R., Karney, B. R., Osilla, K. C., Burns, R. M., & Calderone, L. B. (2008). *Prevalence of PTSD, depression, and TBI among returning service members. In Invisible Wounds of War*. Santa Monica: RAND Corporation.

Report, M. S. M. (2007). Update: Deployment health assessments, U.S. Armed Forces, January 2003–November 2007. *AMSA Medical Surveillance Monthly Report, 14*(8), 12–25.

Ricci, J. A., & Chee, E. (2005). Lost productive time associated with excess weight in the U.S. workforce. *Journal of Occupational and Environmental Medicine, 47*(12), 1227–1234.

Riviere, L. A., & Merrill, J. C. (2011). The impact of combat deployment on military families. In A. B. Adler, P. D. Bliese, & C. A. Castro (Eds.), *Deployment psychology*. Washington, DC: American Psychological Association.

Roy, T. C., Springer, B. A., McNulty, V., & Butler, N. L. (2010). Physical fitness. *Military Medicine, 175*(8), 14–20.

Schneiderman, A. I., Braver, E. R., & Kang, H. K. (2008). Understanding sequelae of injury mechanisms and mild traumatic brain injury incurred during the conflicts in Iraq and Afghanistan: Persistence of postconcussive symptoms and posttraumatic stress disorder. *American Journal of Epidemiology, 167*, 1446–1452.

Seal, K. H., Bertenthal, D., Miner, C. R., Sen, S., & Marmar, C. (2007). Bringing the war back home: Mental health disorders among 103,788 veterans returning from Iraq and Afghanistan seen at Department of Veterans Affairs facilities. *Archives of Internal Medicine, 167*(5), 476–482.

Service, P. H. (1991). *Health people 2000: National health promotion and disease prevention objectives—Full report, with commentary (DHHS Publication No. PHS 91–50212)*. Washington, DC: U.S. Department of Health and Human Services.

Smith, T. C., Zamorski, M., Smith, B., Riddle, J. R., LeardMann, C. A., Wells, T. S., et al. (2007). The physical and mental health of a large military cohort: Baseline functional status of the Millenium Cohort. *BMC Public Health, 7*, 340.

Stahre, M. A., Brewer, R. D., Fonseca, V. P., & Naimi, T. S. (2009). Binge drinking among U.S. active-duty military personnel. *American Journal of Preventive Medicine, 36*(3), 208–217.

Stewart, W. F., Ricci, J. A., Chee, E., & Morganstein, D. (2003). Lost productive work time costs from health conditions in the United States: Results from the American Productivity Audit. *Journal of Occupational and Environmental Medicine, 45*(12), 1234–1246.

Thompson, M. M., & McCreary, D. R. (2006). Enhancing mental readiness in military personnel. In: Alder, A. B., Castro, C. A., & Britt, T. (Eds.), *Military life: The psychology of serving in peace and combat: Vol. 2. Operational stress*. Westport, CT: Praeger.

USA Today (2011, November 30). Troops with PTSD straining resources. By Greg Zoroya.

U.S. Department of the Army. (2012). *Army 2020: Generating health and discipline in the force ahead of the strategic reset*. Washington, DC: Department of the Army.

Vinokur, A. D., Pierce, P. F., Lewandowski-Romps, L., Hobfoll, S. E., & Galea, S. (2011). Effects of war exposure on air force personnel's mental health, job burnout and other organizational related outcomes. *Journal of Occupational Health Psychology, 16*(1), 3–17.

Zouris, J. M., Wade, A. L., & Magno, C. P. (2008). Injury and illness casualty distributions among U.S. Army and Marine Corps personnel during Operation Iraqi Freedom. *Military Medicine, 173*, 247–252.

Chapter 2
Methodology

2.1 Overview

This chapter describes the methodology for the 1980–2008 Department of Defense (DoD) Surveys of Health Related Behaviors Among Active Duty Military Personnel (HRB surveys). It includes an overview of the survey series, the sampling design, instrumentation, data collection procedures, and survey performance rates. In addition, this chapter describes the military respondents and sociodemographic characteristics of the military, and provides an overview of measurement approaches and analysis techniques used throughout this book. The similarity of the study design and consistency of measures over the years permit comparisons of estimates across the surveys. Furthermore, the similarity of key DoD survey measures to those used in civilian surveys enables comparisons of some measures across military and civilian populations.

2.2 Sampling Design

The HRB surveys from 1980 to 2005 followed a nonreplacement sampling approach. For these surveys, the target population consisted of all active duty military personnel in the Army, Navy, Marine Corps, and Air Force except recruits, service academy students, persons absent without official leave, and persons who had a permanent change of station at the time of data collection. These latter personnel were excluded because they either were not accessible or were not on active duty long enough to typify the services. Although personnel who had a permanent change of station are typical of military personnel, they were excluded from the target population because of the practical difficulties of obtaining data from them quickly enough to be of use to the study. It was assumed that the substance use and health behaviors for these individuals were similar to those of other personnel represented in the survey.

R.M. Bray et al., *Understanding Military Workforce Productivity: Effects of Substance Abuse, Health, and Mental Health*, DOI 10.1007/978-0-387-78303-1_2, © Springer Science+Business Media New York 2014

The 2008 HRB survey used a replacement sampling approach and expanded its scope to include the U.S. Coast Guard. Thus, the target population included all Army, Navy, Marine Corps, Air Force, and Coast Guard personnel who were on active duty at the time of data collection except recruits and academy cadets. Replacement sampling was used for persons who were not accessible at the time of data collection due to deployments, temporary duty assignments, leave, transfers, hospitalization/illness, incarceration, or being absent without leave, deceased, unknown at the installation, or separated from service. Personnel inaccessible for these reasons were replaced with a person of the same pay grade and gender taken from the replacement sample or, if the replacement list was exhausted (e.g., due to a high number of deployments), from names on the current personnel rosters of the same pay grade and gender. Replacements were never made for sample members who were available at the installation but chose not to answer the survey. To maintain comparability with prior surveys, Coast Guard data for the 2008 survey were omitted from the analyses presented in this book. Coast Guard analyses appear in the final report for the 2008 HRB survey (Bray et al., 2009) and in a special Coast Guard report (Bray et al., 2011).

The sampling frame (i.e., a comprehensive list of active duty military personnel) was constructed using data provided by the military services during the early years of the survey and from Defense Manpower Data Center during the survey's later years. The sampling frame generally consisted of clustering personnel around military installations where they could be surveyed in large groups. A two-stage probability design was used. The first stage was to select a random sample of approximately 60 military installations from the frame (30 in 2002 due to changes in command activities after the attacks of September 11, 2001) located worldwide, stratified by service (Army, Navy, Marine Corps, Air Force) and region. Region strata varied over the survey years. The 1980 survey used four regions: Continental United States (CONUS), Europe, Pacific, and Other; the 1982–1992 surveys used four slightly modified regions: Americas, North Pacific, Other Pacific, Europe; and the 1995–2008 surveys used two regions: CONUS and Outside the Continental United States (OCONUS). The reason for the change from four regions to two regions in 1995 was to reflect the shifting distribution of the location of the U.S. military forces due to the military drawdown in size and the reassignment of many overseas personnel back to CONUS. The 2005 and 2008 surveys also included a remote stratum to better identify persons who were not located close to a major installation. In 2008, samples were drawn within major commands chosen by the military instead of simply within each service branch. For adequate representativeness, at least two installations per command were selected. In the 2008 survey, 64 installations were selected for the study.

In the second stage, active duty personnel, stratified by pay grade and gender, were randomly selected at the participating installations (and for 2005 and 2008 from the remote stratum). Military pay grade for enlisted personnel was grouped in ascending order of rank as E1–E3 (junior enlisted), E4–E6 (middle enlisted), and E7–E9 (senior enlisted). Pay grades for officers and warrant officers were grouped as O1–O3 (junior officers), O4–O10 (senior officers), and W1–W5 (warrant officers). Officers and women were oversampled because of their smaller numbers. A primary objective of the sampling design was to facilitate the planned on-site group administration of the survey questionnaire to military personnel selected to represent the military in the survey. Because of the worldwide geographic distribution of active duty military personnel, a dual-mode sampling design was developed that called for the survey instrument to be group-administered at large installations, including aboard afloat ships (where hundreds of personnel could be assembled), and mailed to persons in smaller locations where it was not practical to conduct on-site group sessions. Additional details on the sampling procedures and sampling design are contained in survey-specific reports (Bray et al., 1983, 1986, 1988, 1992, 1995, 1999, 2003, 2006, 2009; Burt, Biegel, Carnes, & Farley, 1980).

2.3 Survey Instrumentation and Data Collection Procedures

2.3.1 Survey Questionnaires

For all of the surveys, the instrument was a self-administered paper-and-pencil questionnaire designed for optical-mark reader scanning. All surveys assessed the prevalence of alcohol use, illicit drug use, and tobacco use, as well as adverse consequences associated with substance use. Over the years, the scope of the survey items has broadened. Beginning in 1985, the surveys started to assess the effects of health behaviors other than substance use on the quality of life of military personnel. In 1988, this was expanded in line with DoD health promotion objectives to include information about knowledge of and attitudes toward acquired immunodeficiency syndrome (AIDS). In 1992, the survey was broadened further to give greater emphasis to nutrition and health risks and knowledge and beliefs about AIDS transmission. The 1992 survey also examined other special issues, including the impact of Operations Desert Shield and Desert Storm on substance use rates and the effects of problem gambling in the military.

In 1995, the health behavior questions were revised and items added to assess selected *Healthy People 2000* objectives; the mental health of the force; and specific health concerns of military women, including stress, pregnancy, substance use during pregnancy, and receipt of health services. In 1998, the health behavior questions were revised and items added to assess oral health, men's health, and gambling behavior. The 2002 survey was revised to reflect the continuing need for the services to better understand substance use and mental health issues. Specifically, the assessment of alcohol dependence was broadened to reflect symptomatology consistent with diagnostic criteria from the *Diagnostic and Statistical Manual of Mental Disorders* (*DSM-IV*) (American Psychiatric Association [APA], 1994), and items were added to assess selected *Healthy People 2010* objectives, risk-taking and impulsiveness, reasons for limiting drinking, spiritual practices, anxiety, suicide ideation, and expectancies or beliefs about smoking. In 2005, revisions were made to the alcohol use items to be consistent with items from the Alcohol Use Disorders Identification Test (AUDIT), questions were added to assess nicotine dependence, questions on illicit drug use were revised to add descriptions of drug use categories, and questions were added on sexual enhancers. In addition, questions were added to better assess nutrition and overweight, use of complementary or alternative medicine treatments, serious mental illness, suicide attempts, and deployment and its effects.

The questionnaire for the 2008 survey was patterned after the 2005 questionnaire but broadened to include more information about deployment, combat experiences, mild traumatic brain injury, and mental health issues. Specifically, it included a broad array of items about the following:

- Problems and context associated with alcohol use
- Reasons for drinking and limiting drinking
- Use of cigarettes and other forms of tobacco
- Reasons for starting to smoke cigarettes, intentions to quit smoking, and actual attempts to quit
- Items about nonmedical use of drugs other than alcohol and tobacco that incorporated some wording changes and more complete information on prescription drug misuse (see Sect. 2.7.1)
- Health behaviors related to exercise and nutrition
- Injuries and use of seatbelts and helmets
- Stress experienced at work or in family life, specific sources of stress, and coping behaviors
- Combat exposure experiences
- Deployment experiences (number, type, injuries, length)
- Mild traumatic brain injury
- Mental well-being with an emphasis on screeners suggesting need for further evaluation for depression, serious psychological distress, generalized anxiety disorder, posttraumatic stress disorder (PTSD), and physical and sexual abuse
- Special topics, such as sexual health, gender-specific issues, oral health, gang involvement, and hearing protection
- Job satisfaction

2.3.2 *Data Collection*

Most military personnel completed the questionnaire during group sessions conducted by field teams at the installations where they were stationed (e.g., 97 % in 2008), and the rest completed the questionnaire by mail. A Service Liaison Officer (SLO) was appointed for each service, and an Installation Liaison Officer (ILO) was appointed at each participating installation to coordinate survey activities. SLOs informed the services and the installations about the survey, obtained ILO names and contact information, and worked with research teams to coordinate survey scheduling across installations for their service. The ILOs coordinated with commands at the bases and the research teams, arranged rooms for the survey sessions, notified personnel about the survey, and scheduled them into survey sessions.

Two-person trained field teams conducted the survey sessions at the participating installations. At the group sessions, field teams described the purpose of the study, assured participants of anonymity, informed participants of the voluntary nature of the survey, and showed personnel the correct procedures for marking the questionnaire. Team members then distributed the optical-mark questionnaires to participants, who completed and returned them. On average, questionnaires required 50–55 min to complete. During the visit to an installation, team members attempted to survey all eligible individuals. Team members used rosters on laptop computers to document attendance or reasons for absences. Eligible personnel who failed to attend their scheduled session were contacted and asked to attend a subsequent session. At the completion of the site visit, field teams inventoried completed questionnaires, reconciled the inventory with documented counts from the lists of sampled personnel completing the survey, and packaged and shipped the questionnaires for optical-scan processing.

Survey materials were mailed to eligible personnel who did not participate in a session at the installations and personnel who were at a location too remote to attend a session in person. These personnel were sent a packet that included a cover letter explaining the purpose and importance of the study, an introductory handout explaining the study and each participant's rights, a blank questionnaire, and a business reply envelope to use in mailing the completed questionnaire for scanning. Respondents completed the questionnaire anonymously.

2.4 Sample Size and Survey Performance Rates

Performance rate information is useful for assessing the quality of survey field operations and any nonresponse bias that may exist in the data. In this section, we examine sample size along with the eligibility rate and the response rates over the 28-year survey period.

2.4.1 Sample Size

All of the surveys have large samples to permit analyses to be conducted both at the DoD level and among the participating services. As shown in Table 2.1, sample sizes (usable interviews) ranged from 12,756 in 2002 (a lower number due to intensity of preparations for post-9/11 military operations) to 24,690 in 2008.

2.4.2 Eligibility/Accessibility Rates

The eligibility/accessibility rate was defined as the rate at which those individuals who had been selected when the sample was drawn were still present at the

Table 2.1 Survey response data and performance rates for service members in the active component, 1980–2008

| | Year of active duty survey | | | | | | | | | | |
	1980	1982	1985	1988	1992	1995	1998	2002	2005	2008
Response data										
Sample	19,582	26,964	25,547	26,526	25,887	27,141	36,806	29,787	40,000	39,800
Eligibles	16,355	25,844	22,702	23,701	21,220	23,250	29,253	22,956	30,664	35,219
Usable interviews	15,268	21,936	17,328	18,673	16,395	16,193	17,264	12,756	16,146	24,690
Performance rates										
Eligibility/accessibility rate	83.5	95.8	88.9	89.4	82.0	85.7	79.5	77.1	77.9	69.6
Response rate	93.0	84.3	80.4	81.4	77.3	69.6	59.0	55.6	51.8	70.1

Source: DoD Survey of Health Related Behaviors Among Active Duty Military Personnel, 1980–2008

Note: Response data are frequencies; performance rates are percentages. Eligibility/accessibility rates are percentages of sampled military personnel who were still eligible for the study at the time of data collection. Response rates are shown as percentages of eligible personnel who completed the survey. Data for 2008 omit the Coast Guard.

installations several months later when data collection took place. For the surveys from 1980 to 2005, individuals who were initially selected were considered ineligible during data collection if they had already left the military, were absent without leave, were deceased, had been transferred to a different duty location, or had an unknown status. In 2008, eligibility was defined as all active duty personnel except recruits, academy cadets, and personnel who were absent without leave or incarcerated. Using replacement sampling, we were able to replace most of those who would have been considered ineligible in the prior rounds of the survey. In the 2008 survey, we called this the accessibility rate, which was comparable to the eligibility rate for earlier surveys.

The eligibility/accessibility rate can be an important determinant of statistical efficiency because sampling variances are higher when eligibility/accessibility rates are low. If the eligibility/accessibility status is not known for every case, some potential for bias due to missing data is introduced. As shown in Table 2.1, the eligibility/accessibility rate across survey years has been relatively high (over 80 % for 6 of the 10 surveys) and ranges from a high of 96 % (1982) to a low of 70 % (2008). The eligibility/accessibility rates were somewhat lower for the surveys from 1998 to 2008 than for earlier years. The two key factors that account for this are longer periods to conduct the data collection due to resistance from some installations about supporting the survey (hence older, more out-of-date personnel lists toward the end of the field period) and greater troop movements due to increased military operations associated with the conflicts in Afghanistan and Iraq.

2.4.3   Response Rates

The response rate was defined as the rate at which usable questionnaires were obtained across the combined in-person and mail components of data collection. For these calculations, ineligible/inaccessible individuals were excluded (i.e., personnel who were separated, deceased, absent without leave, transferred to another duty location, or of unknown status). Group sessions were much more effective than mail for obtaining usable questionnaires (e.g., 97 % in 2008).

As shown in Table 2.1, response rates ranged from a high of 93 % to a low of 52 % across survey years. Note that response rates were the lowest from 1998 through 2005, but replacement sampling resulted in an improved response rate for 2008. The pattern of decreasing response rates has also been observed for recurring civilian surveys (Groves & Cooper, 1998). Although not shown in the table, response rates also varied substantially with respect to gender (women higher than men), rank (officers higher than enlisted), and service (Air Force higher than other branches). As a result, the respondent distribution was composed of too many women, officers, and members of the Air Force when compared to the original population distribution. These differential response-rate patterns combined with differential answer patterns to the questionnaire represent a potential for nonresponse bias. For example, an estimate of the prevalence of drug use among junior enlisted personnel would be biased if a greater percentage of military women responded to the survey and reported lower levels of drug use than military men. To partially address this, the data for each survey were weighted to represent the population of eligible active duty personnel, and adjustments were made for the potential biasing effects of differential nonresponse.

Post-stratification methods were used to develop the nonresponse adjustment factors. Updated counts of military personnel were obtained from personnel records at Defense Manpower Data Center, and observed eligibility rates were applied to these new personnel counts for the 96 sampling strata defined by the intersection of service, region, gender, and pay grade groups. (Some strata were collapsed due to small sample sizes.) Adjustment factors were then calculated and applied to the weights to correct for differences in the proportion responding in the sample relative to the proportion in the population. Detailed information regarding the characteristics of nonrespondents is limited. Investigation of reasons for nonresponse and survey participation across pay grade groups suggests that respondents appear to be representative of active duty military personnel based on the characteristics used to weight the survey. Differences between respondents and nonrespondents are assumed to be random.

2.5 Survey Participants and Military Population Characteristics

Table 2.2 displays the distribution of HRB survey respondents by sociodemographic characteristics for each of the survey years. The number of respondents is a function of the number of personnel sampled in each service and the response rates. As can be seen in Table 2.2, most subgroups were well represented and had over 1,000 participants; many had several thousand respondents. The smallest subgroup of respondents for all of the surveys was warrant officers (W1–W5) who comprise only about 1 % of the active duty population. These distributions reflect the sampling scheme that selected personnel proportional to their representation in the population, the varying response rates within selected groups, and oversampling of some groups (i.e., officers and women).

Table 2.3 presents the estimated sociodemographic characteristics of active duty military personnel across the survey years. These estimates are based on data from the sample respondents that were weighted and post-stratified to represent the survey-eligible population. As shown in Table 2.3, there have been some changes over the years in the demographic composition of the military. For gender, the percentage of women increased approximately 60 % from 9 % in 1980 to 14 % in 2008. The most notable increase occurred from 1985 to 1992, and the percentage was relatively steady through 2008. The distribution of race/ethnicity has shifted toward fewer white non-Hispanics (71 % in 1980 to 64 % in 2008) to more Hispanics (5 % in 1980 to 10 % in 2008) and "Others" (6 % in 1980 to 9 % in 2008). African American representation has ranged from 17 to 21 % across the time period and was

Table 2.2 Distribution of active duty respondents across survey years, by sociodemographic characteristics, 1980–2008

Sociodemographic characteristic	Year of active duty survey									
	1980	1982	1985	1988	1992	1995	1998	2002	2005	2008
Gender										
Male	13,924	19,874	15,768	16,582	14,447	13,219	13,296	9,506	12,119	17,939
Female	1,344	2,062	1,560	2,091	1,948	2,974	3,968	3,250	4,027	6,751
Race/ethnicity										
White non-Hispanic	10,794	15,618	12,528	12,959	11,284	11,121	11,133	8,594	9,855	14,660
African American non-Hispanic	2,870	3,663	2,928	3,455	3,010	2,671	3,130	2,596	2,633	4,074
Hispanic	702	1,514	1,161	1,494	1,228	1,336	1,829	909	2,004	3,524
Other	886	1,141	710	766	873	1,065	1,172	657	1,654	2,432
Education										
High school or less	8,245	11,209	8,456	8,011	4,627	5,104	4,520	4,072	4,309	7,140
Some college	4,641	7,370	6,013	7,040	7,726	7,035	7,844	5,647	7,023	11,533
College graduate or higher	2,397	3,356	2,842	3,623	4,042	4,054	4,900	3,037	4,814	6,017
Age										
20 or younger	3,252	5,023	2,998	2,577	667	1,605	1,553	1,557	1,298	2,610
21–25	5,374	7,809	6,117	5,677	2,527	3,703	3,940	3,579	4,300	7,753
26–34	4,245	6,120	5,268	6,424	5,978	4,407	5,157	3,415	4,312	7,613
35 or older	2,382	2,983	2,946	3,996	7,223	6,478	6,614	4,205	6,236	6,714
Family status[a]										
Not married	7,102	10,596	4,869	4,925	4,406	5,513	6,399	5,364	6,138	10,796
Married	7,957	11,285	12,357	13,645	11,957	10,667	10,865	7,392	9,844	13,646
Married, spouse not present	1,150	1,992	1,579	1,237	1,048	891	1,314	624	1,265	1,982
Married, spouse present	6,807	9,293	10,778	12,408	10,909	9,776	9,551	6,768	8,579	11,664

(continued)

Table 2.2 (continued)

Sociodemographic characteristic	Year of active duty survey									
	1980	1982	1985	1988	1992	1995	1998	2002	2005	2008
Pay grade										
E1–E3	4,153	7,107	4,904	3,921	1,221	3,114	2,875	2,516	2,593	5,394
E4–E6	7,665	10,354	8,421	9,691	6,746	5,016	6,251	5,183	6,376	11,524
E7–E9	1,252	1,623	1,508	1,942	4,893	4,401	3,882	2,544	3,221	2,924
W1–W5	168	219	156	187	581	632	659	392	399	578
O1–O3	1,267	1,777	1,508	1,793	1,164	1,373	1,779	1,189	1,444	2,443
O4–O10	763	856	832	1,139	1,790	1,657	1,818	932	2,113	1,827
Total personnel	15,268	21,936	17,328	18,673	16,395	16,193	17,264	12,756	16,146	24,690

Source: DoD Survey of Health Related Behaviors Among Active Duty Military Personnel, 1980–2008

Note: Table entries are the number of respondents who completed a usable questionnaire. Data for 2008 omit the Coast Guard.

[a]Estimates by family status beginning in 1998 are not strictly comparable to those from previous survey years. Personnel who reported that they were living as married in 1998, 2002, 2005, and 2008 were classified as "not married." Before 1998, the marital status question did not distinguish between personnel who were married and those who were living as married.

Table 2.3 Sociodemographic characteristics of eligible participant population for active duty military personnel, 1980–2008

Sociodemographic characteristic	Year of active duty survey									
	1980	1982	1985	1988	1992	1995	1998	2002	2005	2008
Gender										
Male	91.2	90.6	91.0	88.8	85.0	87.6	86.3	83.1	85.2	85.7
Female	8.8	9.4	9.0	11.2	15.0	12.4	13.7	16.9	14.8	14.3
Race/ethnicity										
White non-Hispanic	70.7	71.2	72.3	69.4	66.9	67.7	64.5	67.3	64.4	64.0
African American non-Hispanic	18.8	16.7	16.9	18.5	19.9	17.2	17.6	20.7	17.6	16.7
Hispanic	4.6	6.9	6.7	8.0	8.0	8.5	10.8	7.1	8.8	10.4
Other	5.8	5.2	4.1	4.1	5.2	6.6	7.1	5.0	9.2	8.9
Education										
High school or less	54.0	51.1	48.8	42.9	39.0	36.8	31.3	36.0	33.9	32.8
Some college	43.9	30.4	33.6	37.7	37.7	41.9	46.3	44.3	44.1	45.0
College graduate or higher	15.7	15.3	16.4	19.4	19.1	19.3	22.4	19.7	22.0	22.3
Age										
20 or younger	21.3	22.9	17.3	13.8	9.9	11.8	10.2	13.8	14.1	14.7
21–25	35.2	35.6	35.3	30.4	29.2	32.0	28.4	32.9	32.6	32.2
26–34	27.8	27.9	30.4	37.1	37.2	33.2	34.4	28.8	30.3	29.3
35 or older	15.6	13.6	17.0	18.8	23.6	23.1	27.0	24.5	23.1	23.8
Family status[a]										
Not married	47.2	48.8	43.9	39.4	37.5	39.7	39.9	44.3	45.8	45.7
Married	52.8	51.2	56.1	60.6	62.5	60.3	60.1	55.7	54.1	54.3
Married, spouse not present	6.6	7.0	6.8	5.5	6.0	5.3	6.2	4.9	6.3	8.4
Married, spouse present	46.2	44.2	49.3	55.1	56.5	54.9	53.9	50.8	47.8	46.0
Pay grade										
E1–E3	27.2	32.4	28.3	21.0	18.1	21.7	18.9	22.0	24.0	21.0
E4–E6	50.2	47.2	48.6	51.9	55.7	52.2	52.5	51.9	49.6	51.7
E7–E9	8.2	7.4	8.7	10.4	10.4	10.4	10.8	10.8	9.7	10.2
W1–W5	1.1	1.0	0.9	1.0	1.0	1.0	1.2	1.2	1.0	1.4
O1–O3	8.3	8.1	8.7	9.6	8.9	8.7	9.5	8.3	9.4	9.3
O4–O10	5.0	3.9	4.8	6.1	5.9	5.9	7.2	5.8	6.3	6.4
Total personnel	100.0	100.0	100.0	100.0	100.0	100.0	100.0	100.0	100.0	100.0

Source: DoD Survey of Health Related Behaviors Among Active Duty Military Personnel, 1980–2008

Note: Table displays the percentage of military personnel for each year by sociodemographic characteristic (i.e., table displays column percentages). Percentages may not add to 100 because of rounding. Data for 2008 omit the Coast Guard.

[a]Estimates by family status beginning in 1998 are not strictly comparable to those from previous survey years. Personnel who reported that they were living as married in 1998, 2002, 2005, and 2008 were classified as "not married." Before 1998, the marital status question did not distinguish between personnel who were married and those who were living as married.

at 17 % in 2008. From 1980 to 1998, the active duty force became better educated (persons who were college graduates or higher increased from 16 to 22 %; those with a high school education or less decreased from 54 to 33 %), older (persons 35 or older increased from 16 to 24 %; those 20 or younger decreased from 21 to 15 %), and more likely to be married (from 53 to 60 %). However, from 1998 to 2002, there was a shift in the demographic composition toward having less education and being younger and single. This change was most likely a result of young adults joining the military as a patriotic response to the terrorist attacks of September 11, 2001. From 2002 to 2008, educational level increased with the distribution gradually shifting to the distribution noted in 1998. In 2005 and 2008, the marital status and age distributions remained similar to those in 2002. The military pay grade distribution has remained relatively constant over the years with some slight variations, due to the practice of managing and controlling manpower levels using pay grade billets.

2.6 Background Characteristics

Here and in the following sections, we define and describe the key measures used in subsequent chapters of this book. The measures are organized around our conceptual model presented in Chap. 1. Some of the measures are used in two different contexts—sometimes as outcome measures of interest and sometimes as predictors of other outcomes. Background characteristics consist of three groups of measures: sociodemographic characteristics (gender, age, race/ethnicity, education, family status, the presence of children), psychosocial characteristics (risk-taking, history of physical or sexual abuse, avoidance and active coping, and spirituality), and military conditions (pay grade groups, branch of service, regional location, and deployment and exposure to combat-related events).

2.6.1 Sociodemographic Characteristics

The sociodemographic characteristics include gender, age, race/ethnicity, education, family status, and the presence of children living with service members. Definitions for these characteristics are presented in Table 2.4.

2.6.2 Psychosocial Characteristics

Psychosocial characteristics include risk-taking, history of physical or sexual abuse, avoidance and active coping, and spirituality. Definitions for these characteristics are presented below.

Table 2.4 Definitions of sociodemographic characteristics, 2008

Characteristics	Definition
Gender	Male or female
Age	Current age at the time of the survey: Several analyses present estimates for the age groups 20 or younger, 21–25, 26–34, and 35 or older. Other age groups are used in a few analyses
Race/ethnicity	Personnel were classified into four racial/ethnic groups: white non-Hispanic, African American non-Hispanic, Hispanic, and other (all persons not included in prior three groupings)
Education	The highest level of education attained. Categories included high school or less, some college, and college degree or beyond. Personnel with General Educational Development (GED) certification were classified as high school graduates
Family status	Classification of marital status and spouse presence at the duty location: Categories included not married (personnel living as single, widowed, divorced, or separated); married, spouse not present (those who were legally married and whose spouse was not at the duty location); and married, spouse present (those legally married and living with their spouse). These categories differ slightly from surveys prior to 1998 in that those who were living as married were classified as married personnel instead of single personnel as was done in the earlier surveys. Thus, estimates relating to family status in 1998, 2002, 2005, and 2008 are not strictly comparable to those presented in prior survey years
Presence of children	A single binary item indicated whether military personnel had one or more children living with them

Risk-taking/impulsivity. The 2005 and 2008 surveys assessed risk-taking/impulsivity behavior (Cherpitel, 1999). The risk-taking/impulsivity items included the following: (a) I often act on the spur of the moment without stopping to think, (b) I get a real kick out of doing things that are a little dangerous, (c) you might say I act impulsively, (d) I like to test myself every now and then by doing something a little chancy, and (e) many of my actions seem to be hasty. Each item was scored along a 4-point scale (1 = "not at all," 2 = "a little," 3 = "some," 4 = "quite a lot"), and a mean score (rounded to the next highest integer) was created across items for the scale so that scale items retained the same 4-point integer scale. A dichotomous variable was then created that compared "quite a lot" (high) versus "some, a little, or not at all" (medium/low).

History of physical or sexual abuse. To assess physical and sexual trauma or abuse, the 2005 and 2008 surveys included three items from the *Brief Trauma Questionnaire* (Schnurr, Vielhauer, Weathers, & Findler, 1999). This topic was of concern because of the strong relationship between trauma and poor health behaviors. The first item inquired whether respondents were ever physically punished or beaten by a parent, caretaker, or teacher so that they were very frightened, injured, or thought they would be injured. The second item inquired whether they had ever been attacked, beaten, or mugged. The third item inquired whether anyone had ever forced or pressured the respondent into having some type of unwanted sexual contact. Response items inquired whether the trauma happened before age 18, between age 18 and the time they entered the service, or since entering the service. These items were combined to form a dichotomous measure of a lifetime history of physical or sexual abuse.

Avoidance and active coping. Items for avoidance and active coping were developed specifically for the HRB surveys. Respondents were asked, "When you feel pressured, stressed, depressed, or anxious, how often do you engage in each of the following activities?": Talk to a friend or family member, light up a cigarette, have a drink, say a prayer, exercise or play sports, engage in a hobby, get something to eat, smoke marijuana or use other illegal drugs, think of a plan to solve the problem, think about hurting or killing myself. The possible responses were never, rarely, sometimes, or frequently. These items were factor analyzed to determine dimensionality and possible subscales. These analyses yielded two factors: (a) avoidance coping (smoke a cigarette, have a drink of alcohol, get something to eat, smoke marijuana or use other drugs, think about hurting or killing self) and (b) active coping (think of a plan to solve the problem, engage in a hobby, exercise or play sports, say a prayer, talk to a friend or family member). Mean scores were created for each subset of items suggested by the factor analysis, and these scale scores for active and avoidant coping were entered into the analyses.

Spirituality. Respondents were asked to what extent they agreed with two questions regarding the importance of religious/spiritual beliefs and the degree to which religious/spiritual beliefs influenced their decision-making. Respondents' spirituality was categorized as high if they reported "strongly agree" to both questions, moderate if they reported either "strongly agree" or "agree" to at least one of the questions, and low if they reported either "disagree" or "strongly disagree" to both questions. These items were drawn from those used in the National Survey on Drug Use and Health (NSDUH) (Substance Abuse and Mental Health Services Administration [SAMHSA], 2008).

2.6.3 Military Conditions

Military conditions refer to military-specific features that encompass and define military life. These include pay grade, branch of service, region, and deployment and combat exposure. Definitions for each of these measures are presented below.

Pay Grade. Military pay grades for enlisted personnel were grouped as junior enlisted (E1–E3), middle enlisted (E4–E6), and senior enlisted (E7–E9). Pay grades for commissioned officers and warrant officers were grouped as junior commissioned officers (O1–O3), senior commissioned officers (O4–O10), and warrant officers (W1–W5).

Service. Branches of active military included Army, Navy, Marine Corps, and Air Force.

Region. Geographic locations of the installation where personnel were stationed at the time of the survey were classified as CONUS or OCONUS. Navy personnel assigned to afloat ships were classified as OCONUS.

Deployment and Combat Exposure. Exposure to combat and related circumstances was assessed using a 17-item scale adapted from the Marine Corps (Booth-Kewley, Larson, Highfill-Mcroy, Garland, & Gaskin, 2010) and used in the 2006 DoD Survey of Unit Level Influences on Alcohol and Tobacco Use Among Military Personnel (Brown et al., 2007). These items assessed exposure to incoming fire, mines, improvised explosive devices (IEDs), firing on the enemy, viewing dead bodies or human remains, interaction with enemy prisoners of war, and similar circumstances that may be relevant. Each item asked how many times the respondent had been exposed to a given circumstance; response options were 0= "0 times," 1= "1 to 3 times," 2= "4 to 12 times," 3= "13 to 50 times," and 4= "51 or more times." All items were summed, and the sum score was used to create a categorical combat exposure item where a score equal to zero was considered "deployed but no combat exposure," a score from 1 to 9 was considered "deployed, moderate combat exposure," and a score of 10 or greater was considered "deployed, high combat exposure." A fourth category was added to capture personnel who had not been deployed. These cutoffs were subsequently examined with factor analysis and item-scoring methods that suggest that these categories captured meaningful distinctions between groups of scores.

2.7 Substance Abuse, Health, and Mental Health

Our main intermediate outcomes in the conceptual model discussed in Chap. 1 consist of measures of substance use and related negative effects (illicit drug use, heavy alcohol use, alcohol-related serious consequences, alcohol dependence, cigarette smoking, nicotine dependence), health-related behaviors and conditions (overweight and obesity, illness, and injury), and mental health issues (work or family stress, depression, anxiety, PTSD, suicidal ideation, mental health counseling). Each of these measures is described below, along with several related measures. Analyses of substance use are presented in Chap. 3, health-related behaviors and conditions in Chap. 4, and mental health issues in Chap. 5.

2.7.1 Substance Use

Illicit drug use. In the 2008 survey, illicit drug use was measured in terms of the prevalence of any use of 11 categories of drugs or nonmedical use of prescription drugs. The categories of illicit drugs were marijuana or hashish, cocaine (including crack), hallucinogens (PCP, MDA, MDMA, and other hallucinogens), heroin, methamphetamine, inhalants, or GHB/GBL. The categories of prescription drugs included amphetamines/stimulants, tranquilizers/muscle relaxers, barbiturates/sedatives, or pain relievers. Nonmedical use of prescription-type drugs—or prescription drug misuse—was defined as any use of these drugs "on your own," that is, either without a doctor's prescription, or in greater amounts or more often than prescribed, or for any reasons other than as prescribed, such as for the feelings they caused. Over-the-counter drugs were not included in these measures.

The categories have remained consistent for the most part over the survey years to facilitate examination of trends. No attempt was made to measure quantity (e.g., number of pills) or the size of doses for any of these drugs because most respondents are unable to provide useful information of this type and because of the considerable variation in street drug purity.

Several changes were made to the illicit drug questions in the 2005 and 2008 surveys. In 2005, we added examples of specific drugs in the items. For example, when asking about use of "analgesics or other narcotics," we added the parenthetical explanation "(e.g., prescription pain relievers)." There was a significant increase in the prevalence of illicit drug use from 2002 to 2005, primarily because of an increase in reported prescription drug use between those two surveys. Although this increase was likely due at least partially to an increase in prescription drug use from 2002 to 2005 (Department of the Army, 2010), it is also possible that the increase could be partially due to the increased clarity of the questions, as well as to reporting legitimate medical use of prescription-type drugs. For this reason, in 2008 the questions regarding illegal or street drugs and prescription-type drugs were asked separately, and respondents were instructed not to include legitimate use of prescription-type drugs when responding. To further clarify the questions, in some cases, the common names were used in place of the technical term for the drug categories (e.g., questions were asked about use of "pain relievers" rather than "analgesics"). Additional increases in prescription drug use were also found between 2005 and 2008 as are discussed in Chap. 3. Because of these further improvements in question wording in 2005 and 2008, it is possible that some of the changes observed across survey years for these drugs are due to wording changes rather than drug use changes, especially for prescription drug misuse. Nonetheless, there is corroborating evidence of concerns about increases in prescription drug use in the military (Department of the Army, 2010, 2012).

To estimate the prevalence of use, questions were included about use of each drug type (both use of illegal drugs and nonmedical use of prescription drugs) within the past 30 days, within the past 12 months, and in the lifetime. Analyses presented in this book use measures of illicit drug use in the past 30 days. Indices were constructed for illicit drug use categories (e.g., any illicit drug use including prescription drug misuse, any illicit drug use excluding prescription drug misuse, any prescription drug misuse) by creating use/no use dichotomies for each drug category. The measures of illicit drug use and prescription drug misuse are similar to the definitions that have been commonly used in reports based on NSDUH (e.g., SAMHSA, 2011).

Heavy alcohol use. A drinking-level classification scheme was adapted from Mulford and Miller (1960) based on the quantity of alcohol consumed and the frequency of drinking. The quantity per typical drinking occasion and the frequency of drinking for the type of beverage (beer, wine, or hard liquor) with the largest amount of absolute alcohol per day were used to fit individuals into one of 10 quantity/

frequency categories. These categories were then collapsed into five drinking-level groups: abstainers, infrequent/light drinkers, moderate drinkers, moderate/heavy drinkers, and heavy drinkers. Heavy alcohol use, the category of most concern, was defined as drinking five or more drinks per typical drinking occasion at least once a week in the 30 days before the survey. The criterion of five or more drinks to define heavy drinkers is consistent with the approach used in other national surveys of civilians, such as NSDUH (SAMHSA, 2011) and the Monitoring the Future (MTF) study (e.g., Johnston, O'Malley, Bachman, & Schulenberg, 2011) and by the National Institute on Alcohol Abuse and Alcoholism. Even though all of these studies use five or more drinks as a foundation, the definitions vary slightly. NSDUH asks about five or more drinks on five or more days in the past month, whereas the HRB measure assesses five or more drinks at least once a week in the past month, and the MTF asks about five or more drinks in the past two weeks.

Alcohol-related serious consequences. Alcohol-related *serious consequences* refers to the occurrence of one or more of the following problems in the past 12 months: (a) being passed over for promotion because of drinking, (b) receiving a lower score on a performance rating because of drinking, (c) loss of 1 week or more from duty because of a drinking-related illness, (d) Uniform Code of Military Justice (UCMJ) punishment because of drinking, (e) arrest for driving under the influence of alcohol (DUI), (f) alcohol-related arrest other than DUI, (g) alcohol-related incarceration, (h) alcohol-related injury to service member, (i) alcohol-related accident resulting in someone else's injury or property damage, (j) physical fights while drinking, (k) spouse threatening to leave or having left because of drinking, or (l) spouse asking the service member to leave or the service member having left because of drinking.

Symptoms of alcohol dependence. Several different measures of alcohol dependence have been used over the years. These have been based on a Rand Air Force study definition (Polich & Orvis, 1979), the criteria specified in the *DSM-IV* (APA, 1994), and, most recently in 2005 and 2008, the AUDIT. In this book, we report on possible alcohol dependence using the AUDIT, which was developed by the World Health Organization (WHO) as an easy set of questions to screen for excessive drinking and to help guide possible intervention efforts. The AUDIT consists of 10 questions, each scored 0–4, which are summed to yield a total score ranging from 0 to 40. Scores of 20 or above warrant further diagnostic evaluation for possible alcohol dependence.

Cigarette use. Although the surveys examined several types of tobacco use, analyses in this book focus on cigarette smoking in the past month. Current cigarette smokers were defined as those who had smoked at least 100 cigarettes during their lifetime and who last smoked a cigarette during the past 30 days.

Nicotine dependence. Nicotine dependence was assessed using the Fagerstrom Nicotine Dependency Assessment (Heatherton, Kozlowski, & Frecker, 1991), which consists of a six-item scale that has been widely used and validated to assess severity of smoking. Heatherton and colleagues' method scored four of the items 0 or 1 and two of the items 0–3, resulting in a total score ranging from 0 to 10. Persons with scores of 5 or higher were considered to have significant dependence. We followed this same initial scoring, but then collapsed the 10-point scale into a dichotomous indicator (0, 1) where those scoring 5 or higher were set to 1 (significant dependence) and those scoring 4 or lower were set to 0 (low to moderate dependence).

2.7.2 Health-Related Behaviors and Conditions

Beginning in the mid-1980s, the HRB surveys were broadened to include health behaviors other than use of alcohol, illicit drugs, or tobacco. During the transition into the twenty-first century, progress toward *Healthy People 2000 and 2010* goals for the military was examined. In Chap. 4, we assess progress toward *Healthy People 2010* objectives over a 13-year period using data from the 1995 to 2008 HRB surveys. We consider *Healthy People 2010* objectives related to substance use, weight, exercise, and nutrition. In addition, we examine three intermediate health behavior outcomes: overweight/obesity, illness, and injury. Sleep is a health behavior (defined below) that is included as a control variable in our multivariate models in Chaps. 3, 4, and 5.

Weight. Overweight and obesity were defined in terms of the Body Mass Index (BMI), where BMI is weight (in kilograms) divided by the square of height (in meters). Over the years, there have been several standards proposed for defining overweight and obesity. In the summer of 1998, the National Heart, Lung, and Blood Institute (NHLBI) developed national BMI guidelines for screening for overweight and underweight. These guidelines defined four levels of overweight, regardless of age or gender: (a) overweight (BMI of 25.0–29.9), (b) obesity I (BMI of 30.0–34.9), (c) obesity II (BMI of 35.0–39.9), and (d) extreme obesity (BMI of 40.0 or greater). Underweight was defined as BMI of less than 18.5 for both men and women regardless of age (National Heart, Lung, and Blood Institute [NHLBI], 1998). *Healthy People 2010* sets goals to encourage adults aged 20 years or older, regardless of gender, to maintain a healthy weight, defined as a BMI greater than 18.5 and less than 25.0, with underweight defined by BMI less than 18.5; overweight defined by BMI greater than or equal to 25.0, and obesity defined as BMI greater than or equal to 30.0. In 2005, the Department of Health and Human Services (DHHS) and the Department of Agriculture (USDA) released new *Dietary Guidelines for Americans, 2005* (Department of Health and Human Services/U. S. Department of Agriculture [DHHS/USDA], 2005) that reaffirmed the current national approach to overweight screening using BMI. These guidelines use the same BMI criterion as NHLBI for overweight for persons aged 20 or older (i.e., BMI 25.0 or higher). The current national standards for overweight and obesity use criteria that are consistent with international standards and make a clear distinction between the criteria for adults and those for children and adolescents, who are still growing (Kuczmarski & Flegal, 2000). For persons aged 2–19, overweight is calculated using gender-based BMI for age tables based on growth curves for each gender from the Centers for Disease Control and Prevention (CDC). Persons at or over the 95th percentile for their growth curve are classified as overweight.

Although several weight standards have been proposed in recent years, they are generally in agreement about the BMI level for defining overweight and obesity. The main difference is the approach for classifying persons under 20 years of age. In this book, we follow the approach recommended by NHLBI and *Healthy People 2010* to classify all military personnel regardless of age using the same BMI levels: underweight=BMI<18.5; normal or healthy weight=BMI 18.5–24.9; overweight=BMI 25.0–29.9; obese=BMI 30.0 or higher. Our analyses focus on overweight and obesity as well as healthy weight.

Physical Exercise. The 1995 through 2008 HRB surveys included measures of physical exercise as an indicator of fitness. The 1995 through 2002 questions asked respondents to report how often during the past 30 days they (a) ran, jogged, biked, or briskly walked or hiked for 20 min or more or (b) engaged for 20 min or more in other strenuous physical activity such as handball, soccer, racquet sports, or swimming laps. Persons who reported engaging in activities for one or both of these items three or more times per week were classified as meeting the vigorous exercise standard. In 2005 and 2008, the item was modified to more clearly match the wording used in *Healthy People 2010*, and two levels of exercise were indicated: moderate and vigorous. Activity levels were defined with examples. Moderate physical activity included walking briskly, mowing the lawn, dancing, swimming, or bicycling on level terrain. During moderate physical activity, persons should feel some exertion but should be able to carry on a conversation comfortably. Vigorous physical activity included jogging, mowing the lawn with a nonmotorized push mower, chopping wood, participating in high-impact aerobic dancing, swimming continuous laps, or bicycling uphill. These definitions follow the *Dietary Guidelines for Americans, 2005* (DHHS/USDA, 2005). We combined moderate and vigorous categories for purposes of assessing trends. Thus, for the 2005 and 2008 surveys, personnel were scored as engaging in moderate or vigorous exercise at least 20 min or more three or more times per week, or as engaging in less than moderate or vigorous exercise.

Nutrition. Several HRB surveys have included information on nutrition, but the 2005 survey included an expanded module on food intake, diet, and the use of dietary supplements; some of these measures were also included in 2008 but in less detail. The 2005 data allow a comparison of military personnel's intake of food (by categories) with the recommendations in *Healthy People 2010* and the *Dietary Guidelines for Americans, 2005*. These two documents provide science-based national goals and recommendations to promote health and reduce the risk of chronic disease through a healthier diet. *Healthy People 2010* advised Americans to consume a healthful assortment of varying food types (e.g., fruits, vegetables, grains, dairy, protein). Prior to the latest version of the guidelines, which were published in 2005 while our survey was in the field, Americans were advised to consume three or more servings of fruits and vegetables each day. The 2005 version of the *Dietary Guidelines* increased the recommended intake of fruits and vegetables together to nine servings each day (4.5 cups). The *Healthy People 2010* objectives are more conservative and serve as our comparison standard. In Chap. 4, we examine fruit and vegetable intake of three or more times per day and less than three times per day.

Sleep. A measure of average hours of sleep per night during the past 12 months was included in the 2005 and 2008 surveys. Personnel were classified into three groups: those who received 4 or fewer hours of sleep, those who received 5 or 6 h of sleep, and those who received 7 or more hours of sleep.

Illness in the past 12 months. A single item asked respondents how many times they had had an illness in the past 12 months that kept them from duty for a week or longer. Responses were dichotomized to indicate one or more illnesses versus none.

Injury in the past 12 months. Three items assessed how often respondents were injured from three potential sources. The first item asked about the frequency of injuries or pain that restricted respondents' duty or physical activity for a week or longer. The second item asked about injuries sustained during the course of physical training, whether through accident or overuse. The third item assessed the occurrence of injury, by overuse or accident, during activities other than physical training. A dichotomous injury indicator was created in which any occurrence of any of the three types of injury yielded a positive indication of past 12-month injury.

2.7.3 Mental Health

During the period from 1995 to 2008, the HRB surveys expanded the types of items addressing mental health issues; the most comprehensive set of items were asked in the 2008 survey. Mental health intermediate outcomes for this book included work or family stress, depression, generalized anxiety disorder, PTSD, suicidal ideation, and mental health counseling.

Work or family stress. Separate measures asked about work stress and family stress. Personnel were asked to indicate during the past 12 months how much stress they experienced (a) at work or while carrying out their military duties and (b) in their family life or in a relationship with their spouse, live-in fiancé, boyfriend or girlfriend, or the person they date seriously. Responses were none, a little, some, or a lot. These variables were combined into a single measure and dichotomized into those who reported that they experienced a lot of stress from work or family versus those who experienced some stress, a little stress, or no stress.

Depression. To determine whether personnel were in need of further depression screening, the Version A Burnam depression screen that included one item from the Center for Epidemiologic Studies–Depression Scale (CES-D) (Radloff, 1977) and two items from the Diagnostic Interview Schedule (Robins, Helzer, Croughan, & Ratcliff, 1981) was used. From these items, an index of Need for Further Depression Evaluation was constructed based on reports of both current and extended periods of depression. Personnel were defined as needing further evaluation or assessment if they (a) felt sad, blue, or depressed for 2 weeks or more in the past 12 months *or* (b) reported 2 or more years in their lifetime of feeling depressed and felt depressed "much of the time" in the past 12 months *and* (c) felt depressed on 1 or more days in the past week. This index was based on work by Burnam and colleagues (Burnam, Wells, Leake, & Landsverk, 1988; Rost, Burnam, & Smith, 1993) that showed this screener to have high sensitivity and good positive predictive value for detecting depressive disorder.

Generalized anxiety disorder. To screen for generalized anxiety disorder symptoms, a set of items adapted from the Patient Health Questionnaire (Spitzer, Kroenke, & Williams, 1999) was used. If respondents indicated that they had been feeling nervous, anxious, or on edge or that they had been worrying a lot about different things for several days or more, the analysis examined whether they reported any of the other symptoms. If they reported experiencing three or more symptoms on more than half of the days in the past 30 days, they were considered to meet screening criteria.

Posttraumatic stress disorder. The 2005 and 2008 surveys included the PTSD Checklist–civilian version (Keen, Kutter, Niles, & Krinsley, 2008; Ruggiero, Del Ben, Scotti, & Rabalais, 2003; Weathers, Litz, Huska, & Keane, 1994), which consists of a set of 17 items that ask about experiences related to PTSD. The civilian version was used rather than military version in order to capture PTSD symptoms that may be the result of either military or nonmilitary experiences (i.e., traumatic exposures that occurred before being in the service). Items included characteristics such as loss of interest in activities that used to be enjoyable, being extremely alert or watchful, having physical reactions when reminded of a stressful experience, and feeling jumpy or easily startled. Respondents were asked to indicate how much they had been bothered by each of the 17 items in the past 30 days; response options were not at all, a little bit, moderately, quite a bit, and extremely. Each statement was scored from 1 to 5, and a sum for all items was computed. The standard diagnostic cutoff was used such that if the sum were greater than or equal to 50, participants were classified as needing further evaluation for current (past month) PTSD; those with a score less than 50 were considered not to need further evaluation (Forbes, Creamer, & Biddle, 2001). It should be noted that the published cutpoints used to indicate need for further evaluation of PTSD were derived from samples with high prevalence rates of current PTSD and should be interpreted with caution (Orr & Kaloupek, 2004).

Suicidal ideation. The 2005 and 2008 surveys included questions about suicide contemplation. Items asked whether respondents had seriously considered suicide and, if so, during what time period. A dichotomous variable was created indicating whether active duty service members had seriously considered suicide within the past year.

Mental health counseling. Respondents were asked whether they had received mental health or substance abuse counseling in the past 12 months from any of the following sources: a mental health professional at a military facility; a general medical doctor at a military facility; a military chaplain; a civilian mental health professional; a general medical doctor at a civilian facility; a civilian pastor, rabbi, or other pastoral counselor; or a self-help group. A dichotomous variable was created indicating whether personnel had received any counseling.

2.8 Activity Limitations and Productivity Loss

Activity limitations related to physical and mental health served as two additional intermediate outcomes for the final productivity loss model. These two measures are examined only in Chap. 6 as part of the model and are not elaborated on elsewhere. Productivity loss was our final outcome measure. Unfortunately, our data did not have a direct measure of worker productivity but did have several items regarding decrements in productivity that were used to develop two indicators of productivity loss. Analyses of these measures are also presented in Chap. 6.

2.8.1 Physical Health-Limited Activity

A single item asked respondents how often during the past 30 days poor physical health kept them from doing their usual activities, such as work or recreation. A dichotomous measure was created indicating whether this had occurred on 1 or more days.

2.8.2 Mental Health-Limited Activity

A single item asked respondents how often during the past 30 days poor mental health kept them from doing their usual activities, such as work or recreation. A dichotomous measure was created indicating whether this had occurred on 1 or more days.

2.8.3 Productivity Loss

Productivity loss was measured based on 5 items that asked how many work days in the past 12 months personnel reported any of the following: (a) being late for work by 30 min or more, (b) leaving work early for a reason other than an errand or early holiday leave, (c) being hurt in an on-the-job accident, (d) working below one's normal level of performance, or (e) not coming to work at all because of an illness or a personal accident. Two measures were developed from these five items.

The first measure was a composite indicator in which each of the 5 items was dichotomized to create an indicator of 0 or 1 or more days occurrence. These binary indicators were then summed to create a composite productivity loss measure ranging from 0 to 5. This composite measure was calculated for each of the surveys from 1995 to 2008 and was used to examine the prevalence and trends in productivity loss.

The second measure consisted of using the five productivity loss items to form a latent factor indicator as our final outcome measure of productivity loss. The latent factor was estimated with confirmatory factor analysis and evaluated for fit using the comparative fit index and the root-mean-square error of approximation. These indices showed a good fit for the latent factor of productivity loss. Chapter 6 provides additional details about the development of this final outcome measure.

2.9 Analytical Approach

The goal of the analyses for this book was to examine patterns, trends, and relationships about the productivity loss model components among active duty military personnel. Several types of analyses were conducted:

- Descriptive univariate and bivariate analyses of the prevalence of various health behaviors
- Assessment of trends in various behaviors (e.g., substance use, overweight, stress) from 1980 to 2008 or for the period of years that the data were available
- Standardized comparisons of military and civilian rates of substance use
- Logistic regression analyses
- Structural equation modeling (SEM)

Many of our analyses presented in Chaps. 3–5 were logistic regressions. For these, our approach was to select variables from the categories noted in our conceptual model. We then performed initial analyses to determine the most important variables in the models, generally dropping nonsignificant variables in subsequent iterations to simplify the overall models. We tended to retain sociodemographic and military condition variables in the models, although occasionally some of these were also dropped when we encountered model limitations due to multicollinearity or problematic deficiency in cells (i.e., some categories of a predictor had no variability on the outcome).

An important part of our analyses included the comparison of trends across the series of HRB surveys. Although comparing trends over time is useful, such analyses have limitations. The data from the HRB survey series are cross-sectional, not longitudinal, and come from different populations because of the relatively high turnover among military personnel. Many individuals serving in the military in the 1980s were no longer in the military in 2008. Thus, caution is required when making inferences about reasons for the observed changes in rates of substance use, health behaviors, or mental health problems. The changes may be partly due to effective substance use, health promotion, and mental health programs and other health-related policies in the military, but they also may be due to differences in demographic characteristics, attitudes, and values of the populations being surveyed.

In Chap. 6, we use SEM to relate the various sets of variables from earlier chapters of the book to predict productivity loss. To represent the productivity loss construct, we used the latent factor model of productivity loss described above. In addition, substance use and mental health were modeled as latent factors. Model fit for these confirmatory factor models was good, indicating that these were adequate representatives of the data and composites of the multiple items that made up each dimension. In contrast, the physical health items, such as overweight and illness, did not form a latent variable with adequate fit properties, so these items were entered as individual observed variables. Structural paths were added to the model to reflect the putative causal mechanisms that ultimately lead to productivity loss. The mental health and substance use factors together with overweight, exercise, illness, and injury all were predictors of productivity loss as well as the intermediate outcomes of physical health-limited activities and mental health-limited activities. Thus, for each of the principal predictors of productivity loss (e.g., substance use), two explanatory mechanisms were estimated: the direct impact of the predictor on productivity loss and the impact of the predictor as transmitted through activity limitations.

2.10   Strengths and Limitations of the Data

Self-reports in which service members provide data about their behaviors rely on respondents' veracity and ability to provide correct information about observations and events. Surveys have been a major vehicle for obtaining self-reported data about a wide variety of behaviors, including substance use and health behaviors. A major strength of the HRB surveys is that they have permitted the collection of a rich array of information from active duty service members around the world about the nature and extent of behaviors of interest along with information about correlates of these behaviors. Other strengths of the surveys include large numbers of participants, the use of sophisticated sampling techniques, and questionnaire items that allow for precise estimates of substance use, mental health, and other health behaviors for well-defined populations and that permit assessment of trends over time.

Despite these strengths, survey results are subject to the potential for self-report bias and the ambiguities caused by questions with varying interpretations. In addition, there are other potential problems with the validity of survey data, including issues of population coverage and response rates. If the population is not properly represented in the survey or if response rates are low, biases may be introduced that can invalidate the survey results. The design and field procedures of the HRB surveys addressed these concerns to the extent possible using the most current survey methodology. Questionnaire pretests were used to identify and eliminate ambiguities in question wording. State-of-the-art scientific sampling procedures were used to select a large number of participants who represented the active duty population for each of the services. The questionnaires were administered anonymously and participants were given assurances of data confidentiality by civilian teams to encourage honest reporting, especially on sensitive items. Response rates have been within acceptable ranges given a challenging military environment.

Response rates declined from the late 1990s to 2005 but improved in 2008. Surveys with lower response rates have greater potential for nonresponse bias in the estimates, which means that it is more likely that persons who did not take part may have answered differently (had they taken part) than those who participated. For example, if drug or heavy alcohol users were missed in the survey, then survey estimates of drug use and heavy alcohol use would be underestimates of these behaviors. Unfortunately, because no formal nonresponse studies were conducted, we have no way of addressing this problem directly. However, several bits of evidence suggest that estimates are not likely to have substantial bias. First, a comparison of the rates of nonresponse across pay grades for the surveys showed fairly similar rates, indicating that all pay grade groups were appropriately represented. Second, nonresponse weighting adjustments were made to help compensate for the potential bias of nonsurveyed persons (i.e., the responding population was weighted to represent the broader military population). Third, examination of substance abuse data shows increases in rates of heavy drinking and cigarette use from the 1998 to 2002, which largely remained the same in 2005 and 2008. These increases argue somewhat against seriously biased estimates because such increases would not be expected if substantial numbers of users were missed in the surveys.

Many individuals question the validity of self-reported data on sensitive topics, such as alcohol and drug use, claiming that survey respondents will give socially desirable, rather than truthful, answers. In some situations, respondents may have strong motivations not to report drug use behavior honestly, and data may yield drug use estimates that are conservative. This issue was of concern for the surveys because of the belief that service members might not reveal anything about behaviors that could jeopardize their military careers.

These issues have been the topic of a number of empirical investigations, which have demonstrated that, although self-reports may underestimate the extent of substance use, they generally provide useful and meaningful data. For example, in an examination of the validity of alcohol-problem measures among Air Force personnel, Polich and Orvis (1979) found little evidence of underreporting when comparing self-reported data on adverse effects with police records and supervisor reports. Air Force beverage sales data, however, suggested that self-reports may underestimate the actual prevalence of alcohol use by as much as 20 %.

The reliability and the validity of self-reported data among respondents from the U.S. civilian general population have been tested explicitly in relation to alcohol use (Lemmens, Tan, & Knibbe, 1992; Mayer & Filstead, 1979; Midanik, 1982; Smith, Remington, Williamson, & Anda, 1990) and drug use (Haberman, Josephson, Zanes, & Elinson, 1972; Harrison, 1995; Kandel & Logan, 1984; O'Malley, Bachman, & Johnston, 1983; Rouse, Kozel, & Richards, 1985). Overall, the various reviews of the literature are encouraging in suggesting that self-reports on alcohol use and drug use can be reasonably reliable and valid.

Additional information about the validity of self-reports on drug use has been addressed by Harrison, Martin, Enev, and Harrington (2007), Harrison (1995), and Rouse et al. (1985). One general conclusion emerging from these reviews is that most people appear to be truthful under the proper conditions. Such conditions include believing that the research has a legitimate purpose, having suitable privacy for providing answers, having assurances that answers will be kept confidential, and believing that those collecting the data can be trusted (Harrison, 1995; Johnston & O'Malley, 1985). When respondents believe that survey questions are reasonable and justified in terms of their purpose, and when they have confidence that their answers will not be used against them, self-reports can be sufficiently valid for research and policy purposes. When those conditions are not met, there may be substantial underreporting of substance use.

The validity of the data reported across the HRB surveys is supported by this body of research and the methodological rigor used to conduct the studies. Throughout the HRB survey series, a strong research design has been used, and rigorous procedures have been followed that encourage honest reporting as noted above.

References

American Psychiatric Association. (1994). *Diagnostic and statistical manual of mental disorders* (4th ed.). Washington, DC: Author.

Booth-Kewley, S., Larson, G. E., Highfill-Mcroy, R. M., Garland, C. F., & Gaskin, T. A. (2010). Correlates of posttraumatic stress disorder symptoms in marines back from war. *Journal of Traumatic Stress, 23*(1), 69–77.

Bray, R. M., Guess, L. L., Mason, R. E., Hubbard, R. L., Smith, D. G., & Marsden, M. E., et al. (1983). *1982 worldwide survey of alcohol and non-medical drug use among military personnel* (RTI/2317/01-01F). Report prepared for the Assistant Secretary of Defense (Health Affairs), U.S. Department of Defense. Research Triangle Park, NC: Research Triangle Institute.

Bray, R. M., Hourani, L. L., Rae, K. L., Dever, J. A., Brown, J. M., & Vincus, A. A., et al. (2003). *2002 Department of Defense survey of health related behaviors among military personnel.* Report prepared for the Assistant Secretary of Defense (Health Affairs), U.S. Department of Defense, Cooperative Agreement No. DAMD17-00-2-0057/RTI/7841/006-FR. Research Triangle Park, NC: Research Triangle Institute.

Bray, R. M., Hourani, L. L., Rae Olmsted, K. L., Witt, M., Brown, J. M., Pemberton, M. R., et al. (2006). *2005 Department of Defense survey of health related behaviors among active duty military personnel.* Report prepared for the Assistant Secretary of Defense (Health Affairs), U.S. Department of Defense (RTI/7841/106-FR). Research Triangle Park, NC: Research Triangle Institute.

Bray, R. M., Kroutil, L. A., Luckey, L. W., Wheeless, S. C., Iannacchione, V. G., & Anderson, D. W., et al. (1992). *1992 worldwide survey of substance abuse and health behaviors among military personnel.* Report prepared for the Assistant Secretary of Defense (Health Affairs), U.S. Department of Defense. Research Triangle Park, NC: Research Triangle Institute.

Bray, R. M., Kroutil, L. A., Wheeless, S. C., Marsden, M. E., Bailey, S. L., & Fairbank, J. A., et al. (1995). *1995 Department of defense survey of health related behaviors among military personnel.* Report prepared for the Assistant Secretary of Defense (Health Affairs), U.S. Department of Defense. (DoD Contract No. DASO1-94-C-0140). Research Triangle Park, NC: Research Triangle Institute.

Bray, R. M., Marsden, M. E., Guess, L. L., Wheeless, S. C., Iannacchione, V. G., & Keesling, S. R. (1988). *1988 worldwide survey of substance abuse and health behaviors among military personnel*. Report prepared for the Assistant Secretary of Defense (Health Affairs), U.S. Department of Defense. Research Triangle Park, NC: Research Triangle Institute.

Bray, R. M., Marsden, M. E., Guess, L. L., Wheeless, S. C., Pate, D. K., & Dunteman, G. H., et al. (1986). *1985 worldwide survey of alcohol and nonmedical drug use among military personnel*. Report prepared for the Assistant Secretary of Defense (Health Affairs), U.S. Department of Defense. Research Triangle Park, NC: Research Triangle Institute.

Bray, R. M., Pemberton, M. R., Hourani, L. L., Witt, M., Rae Olmsted, K. L., & Brown, J. M., et al. (2009) *2008 Department of Defense survey of health related behaviors among active duty military personnel*. Report prepared for TRICARE Management Activity, Office of the Assistant Secretary of Defense (Health Affairs) and U.S. Coast Guard. Research Triangle Park, NC: Research Triangle Institute.

Bray, R. M., Rae Olmsted, K. L., Brown, J. M., Witt, M. B., Lane, M. E., & Anderson, E. M., et al. (2011). *State of the behavioral health of the United States Coast Guard*. Report prepared for United States Coast Guard. Research Triangle Park, NC: Research Triangle Institute.

Bray, R. M., Sanchez, R. P., Ornstein, M. L., Lentine, D., Vincus, A. A., & Baird, T. U., et al. (1999). *1998 Department of Defense survey of health related behaviors among military personnel*. Report prepared for the Assistant Secretary of Defense (Health Affairs), U.S. Department of Defense, Cooperative Agreement No. DAMD17-96-2-6021, RTI/7034/006-FR). Research Triangle Park, NC: Research Triangle Institute.

Brown, J. M., Bray, R. M., Calvin S. L., Vandermaas-Peeler, R., Rae Olmsted, K. L., & Ginder, S. A., et al. (2007) *2006 unit level influences on alcohol and tobacco use*. Report prepared for the Assistant Secretary of Defense (Health Affairs), U.S. Department of Defense. Research Triangle Park, NC: Research Triangle Institute.

Burnam, M. A., Wells, K. B., Leake, B., & Landsverk, J. (1988). Development of a brief screening instrument for detecting depressive disorders. *Medical Care, 26*(8), 775–789.

Burt, M. A., Biegel, M. M., Carnes, Y., & Farley, E. C. (1980). *Worldwide survey of non-medical drug use and alcohol use among military personnel: 1980*. Bethesda, MD: Burt Associates.

Cherpitel, C. J. (1999). Substance use, injury, and risk-taking dispositions in the general population. *Alcoholism, Clinical and Experimental Research, 23*(1), 121–126.

Department of Health and Human Services/U. S. Department of Agriculture. (2005). *Dietary guidelines for Americans*. Washington, DC: U.S. Government Printing Office.

Department of the Army. (2010). *Army health promotion risk reduction suicide prevention report*. Washington, DC: Department of the Army.

Department of the Army. (2012). *Army 2020: Generating health and discipline in the force ahead of the strategic reset*. Washington, DC: Department of the Army.

Forbes, D., Creamer, M., & Biddle, D. (2001). The validity of the PTSD checklist as a measure of symptomatic change in combat-related PTSD. *Behaviour Research and Therapy, 39*(8), 977–986.

Groves, R., & Cooper, M. (1998). *Nonresponse in Household Interview Survey*. New York: Wiley.

Haberman, P., Josephson, E., Zanes, A., & Elinson, J. (1972). High school drug behavior: A methodological report on pilot studies. In S. Einstein & S. Allen (Eds.), *Proceedings of the First International Conference on Student Drug Surveys*. Baywood: Farmingdale, NY.

Harrison, L. D. (1995). The validity of self-reported data on drug use. *Journal of Drug Issues, 25*, 91–111.

Harrison, L. D., Marton, S. S., Enev, T., & Harrington, D. (2007). *Comparing drug testing and self-report of drug use among youths and young adults in the general population* (DHHS Publication No. SMA 07-4249, Methodology Series M-7). Rockville, MD: Substance Abuse and Mental Health Services Administration, Office of Applied Studies.

Heatherton, T. F., Kozlowski, L. T., & Frecker, R. C. (1991). The Fagerstrom test for nicotine dependence: a revision of the Fagerstrom Tolerance Questionnaire. *British Journal of Addiction, 86*(9), 1119–1127.

Johnston, L. D. & O'Malley, P. M. (1985). Issues of validity and population coverage in student surveys of drug use. In B. A. Rouse, N. J. Kozel, & L. G. Richards (Eds.), *Self-report methods of estimating drug use: Meeting current challenges to validity* (NIDA Research Monograph 57, DHHS Publication No. ADM 85–1402, pp. 31–54). Rockville, MD: National Institute on Drug Abuse.

Johnston, L. D., O'Malley, P. M., Bachman, J. G., & Schulenberg, J. E. (2011). *Monitoring the Future national survey results on drug use, 1975–2010. Volume II: College students and adults ages 19–50* (NIH Publication No. 09–7403). Bethesda, MD: National Institute on Drug Abuse.

Kandel, D. B., & Logan, J. A. (1984). Patterns of drug use from adolescence to young adulthood: 1. Periods of risk for initiation, continued use and discontinuation. *American Journal of Public Health, 74*, 660–666.

Keen, S. M., Kutter, C. J., Niles, B. L., & Krinsley, K. E. (2008). Psychometric properties of PTSD checklist in sample of male veterans. *Journal of Rehabilitation Research and Development, 45*, 465–474.

Kuczmarski, R. J., & Flegal, K. M. (2000). Criteria for definition of overweight in transition: Background and recommendations for the United States. *American Journal of Clinical Nutrition, 72*, 1074–1081.

Lemmens, P., Tan, E. S., & Knibbe, R. A. (1992). Measuring quantity and frequency of drinking in a general population survey: A comparison of five indices. *Journal of Studies on Alcohol, 53*, 476–486.

Mayer, J., & Filstead, W. J. (1979). The adolescent alcohol involvement scale: An instrument for measuring adolescents' use and misuse of alcohol. *Journal of Studies on Alcohol, 40*, 291–300.

Midanik, L. (1982). The validity of self-reported alcohol consumption and alcohol problems: A literature review. *British Journal of Addiction, 77*, 357–382.

Mulford, H. A., & Miller, D. A. (1960). Drinking in Iowa: 2. The extent of drinking and selected sociocultural categories. *Quarterly Journal of Studies on Alcohol, 21*, 26–39.

National Heart, Lung, and Blood Institute. (1998). *Clinical guidelines on the identification, evaluations, and treatment of overweight and obesity in adults.* Retrieved January 5, 1999, from http://www.nhlbi.nih.gov/nhlbi/cardio/obes/prof/guidelns/ob_home.htm.

O'Malley, P. M., Bachman, J. G., & Johnston, L. D. (1983). Reliability and consistency in self-reports of drug use. *International Journal of the Addictions, 18*, 805–824.

Orr, S. P., & Kaloupek, D. G. (2004). Psychophysiological assessment of posttraumatic stress disorder. In J. P. Wilson & T. M. Keane (Eds.), *Assessing psychological trauma and PTSD* (2nd ed., pp. 69–97). New York: Guilford Press.

Polich, J. M., & Orvis, B. R. (1979). *Alcohol problems: Patterns and prevalence in the U.S. Air Force.* Santa Monica, CA: RAND Corporation.

Radloff, L. S. (1977). The CES-D Scale: A self-report depression scale for research in the general population. *Applied Psychological Measurement, 1*, 385–401.

Robins, L. N., Helzer, J. E., Croughan, J., & Ratcliff, K. S. (1981). National Institute of Mental Health diagnostic interview schedule: Its history, characteristics, and validity. *Archives of General Psychiatry, 38*(4), 381–389.

Rost, K., Burnam, M. A., & Smith, R. (1993). Development of screeners for depressive disorders and substance disorder history. *Medical Care, 31*, 189–200.

Rouse, B. A., Kozel, N. J., & Richards, L. G. (Eds.) (1985). *Self-report methods of estimating drug use: Meeting current challenges to validity* (NIDA Research Monograph 57, DHHS Publication No. ADM 85–1402). Rockville, MD: National Institute on Drug Abuse.

Ruggiero, K. J., Del Ben, K., Scotti, J. R., & Rabalais, A. E. (2003). Psychometric properties of the PTSD checklist—Civilian version. *Journal of Traumatic Stress, 16*, 495–502.

Schnurr, P., Vielhauer, M., Weathers, F., & Findler, M. (1999). *The brief trauma questionnaire.* White River Junction, VT: National Center for PTSD.

Smith, P. F., Remington, P. L., Williamson, D. F., & Anda, R. F. (1990). A comparison of alcohol sales data with survey data on self-reported alcohol use in 21 states. *American Journal of Public Health, 80*, 309–312.

Spitzer, R. L., Kroenke, K., & Williams, J. B. (1999). Validation and utility of a self-report version of PRIME-MD: the PHQ primary care study. Primary Care Evaluation of Mental Disorders. Patient Health Questionnaire. *Journal of the American Medical Association, 282*(18), 1737–1744.

Substance Abuse and Mental Health Services Administration. (2008). *Results from the 2007 National Survey on Drug Use and Health: National Findings* (Office of Applied Studies, NSDUH Series H-34, DHHS Publication No. SMA 08–4343). Rockville, MD: Substance Abuse and Mental Health Services Administration.

Substance Abuse and Mental Health Services Administration. (2011). *Results from the 2010 National Survey on Drug Use and Health: National Findings* (NSDUH Series H-41, HHS Publication No. (SMA) 11–4658). Rockville, MD: Substance Abuse and Mental Health Services Administration, Office of Applied Studies.

Weathers, F. W., Litz, B. T., Huska, J. A., & Keane, T. M. (1994). *The PTSD checklist-civilian version (PCL-C).* Boston, MA: National Center for PTSD.

Chapter 3
Substance Abuse

3.1 Overview and Background

Substance abuse—the problematic or harmful use of illicit drugs, alcohol, and tobacco—is a key influence on lowering the productivity of military personnel and is among the most preventable causes of health- and work-related problems. Illicit drug abuse includes illegal or street drugs such as marijuana, heroin, and cocaine, as well as the nonmedical use of prescription-type drugs. McGinnis, Williams-Russo, and Knickman (2002) maintain that substance abuse is the most important contributor to preventable illnesses, health costs, and related social problems facing the United States today. Further, substance abuse has been called the number one health problem in the country; it places a major burden on health care costs and causes harm to worker productivity, family life, and public safety; it is also responsible for more than one in four deaths each year (Schneider Institute for Health Policy, 2001). In addition, substance abuse is implicated in exposure to human immunodeficiency virus/acquired immunodeficiency syndrome (HIV/AIDS) and other sexually transmitted diseases, motor vehicle crashes, and suicide (Department of Health and Human Services, 2012).

Although some alcohol use may be beneficial in terms of lowering the risk for cardiovascular disease, heavy alcohol use may result in coronary heart disease, cancer, liver cirrhosis, trauma, and other health problems as well as involvement in injury and violence (National Institute on Alcohol Abuse and Alcoholism, 2000). Use of illicit drugs and tobacco may foster impairment in functioning and negative health consequences. Illicit drug use is implicated in cardiovascular disease, stroke, HIV/AIDS, and a host of other medical problems (National Institute on Drug Abuse, 2011a). The effects of smoking on health are well known, and there are no risk-free levels of smoking (Department of Health and Human Services, 2010). Substance use is pervasive. In 2010, 9 % of the civilian population aged 18 or older used illicit drugs, 56 % drank alcohol, 7 % drank heavily, and 24.5 % smoked cigarettes in the past month (Substance Abuse and Mental Health Services Administration, 2011a). Among military personnel in 2008, 12 % used illicit drugs, 78 % drank alcohol,

R.M. Bray et al., *Understanding Military Workforce Productivity: Effects of Substance Abuse, Health, and Mental Health*, DOI 10.1007/978-0-387-78303-1_3,
© Springer Science+Business Media New York 2014

20 % drank heavily, and 31 % smoked cigarettes in the past month (Bray et al., 2010; Bray, Pemberton et al., 2009).

Preventing substance abuse is a cornerstone of *Healthy People 2020* objectives and military health promotion policy. National objectives for improving the health of Americans began with the 1979 Surgeon General's report and have continued to the present. The 1979 report, *Healthy People: The Surgeon General's Report on Health Promotion and Disease Prevention* (U.S. Department of Health, Education, and Welfare, 1979) established ambitious, quantifiable objectives for improving the nation's health by 1990 and emphasized the role of proper nutrition and regular physical exercise in maintaining health. *Healthy People 2020* recognizes that 22 million Americans struggle with drug and alcohol problems and that many are unaware of their problem or do not receive treatment for it. Although progress has been made in lowering the rates of drug and alcohol abuse, the public health toll remains high. Thus, *Healthy People 2020* objectives for substance abuse focus on the priority areas of reducing the percentage of adolescents who use alcohol or illicit drugs and the percentage of adults who smoke cigarettes or engage in binge drinking (Department of Health and Human Services, 2012). Similarly, since the early 1970s, preventing or deterring substance abuse among military personnel has been a focus of the broad Department of Defense (DoD) health promotion policy. Beginning in 1970, DoD established a series of policies and programs to combat drug and alcohol abuse among military personnel, with a policy of zero tolerance toward drug and alcohol abuse (Bray, Marsden, Herbold, & Peterson, 1992; Bray, Marsden, Mazzuchi, & Hartman, 2009; Department of Defense, 1970, 1972, 1980a, 1980b). In 1986, DoD issued a health promotion directive aimed at improving and maintaining military readiness and quality of life (Department of Defense, 1986). This directive included six program areas, two of which were smoking prevention/cessation and alcohol and drug abuse prevention; these areas have continued to be a major focus of military health promotion policy (Bray et al., 2006).

Perhaps related to these national preventive efforts, there have been long-term societal declines in cigarette use and illicit drug use, although the declines in drug use have been accompanied by recent increases. Excessive alcohol use, however, has been more stable. The National Survey on Drug Use and Health (NSDUH) is the nation's primary source of information about the use of illicit drugs, alcohol, and tobacco among members of the U.S. civilian noninstitutionalized population aged 12 and older. Conducted since 1971, trend data from the survey show that the highest rates of marijuana use among younger adults (aged 18–25 and 26–34, ages mirroring the majority of the military population) occurred during the early 1970s to mid-1980s. Rates of this most commonly used illicit drug were lower during the 1990s but have recently increased. For example, rates of past month marijuana use among persons aged 18–25 were 28 % in 1972, 36 % in 1979, 13 % in 1990, 14 % in 2000, and 18 % in 2010 (Substance Abuse and Mental Health Services Administration, 2011a). Among adults aged 18 and older, use of any illicit drugs in the past month has remained fairly constant from 2002 (8 %) to 2010 (almost 9 %). At the same time, rates of binge and heavy drinking were relatively stable among adults aged 18 and older. The rate of binge drinking (five or more drinks on the same occasion on at least 1 day in the past 30 days) was 24 % in 2002 and about

25 % in 2010. The percentage of heavy drinkers (five or more drinks on the same occasion on each of 5 days in the past 30 days) was 7 % in both 2002 and 2010. Past month cigarette use, however, declined in the past decade among adults aged 18 and older, from 28 % in 2002 to 24 % in 2010 (Substance Abuse and Mental Health Services Administration, 2011b). In addition, the National Health Interview Survey found that previous declines in smoking among adults have stalled during the past 5 years; past month cigarette use among adults aged 18 and older was 21 % in both 2005 and 2008 (Centers for Disease Control and Prevention, 2010).

Substance use trends among military personnel mirror generally mirror these civilian trends, although over the past 2 decades the use of illicit drugs has been lower among military personnel than among civilians, use of alcohol has been higher than among civilians, and the use of cigarettes was initially higher in the military, but has gradually converged with civilian rates once demographic differences in the populations are taken into account (Bray, Pemberton et al., 2009; Bray et al., 2010; Bray, Marsden, & Peterson, 1991). Bray and Hourani (2007) traced the changes in substance use among active duty military personnel between 1980 and 2005, documenting declines in cigarette smoking and illicit drug use over that period but less change in heavy alcohol use. They found that these changes could not be explained solely by changes in the demographic composition of the military but possibly to factors such as a military culture supportive of alcohol use and the effects of deployment. Bray, Rae Olmsted, and Williams (2012) found recent increases in prescription drug misuse among military personnel, largely driven by an increase in the misuse of prescription pain medications.

Others have found that the nature of substance use may differ between military personnel and civilians. For example, Ames, Cunradi, and Moore (2002) found that drinking, smoking, and drug use were prevalent among military recruits prior to enlistment. However, rates of heavy drinking were greater among recruits than among the young adult civilian population, while rates of illicit drug use and smoking among recruits were similar to those among the young adult civilian population. According to the National Survey on Drug Use and Health, among veterans and nonveterans in the civilian population, both marijuana use and heavy alcohol use were more prevalent among those who had served in the armed forces than among those who had not; past year alcohol dependence was more prevalent among veterans than nonveterans, while past year illicit drug dependence was the same in both populations (Substance Abuse and Mental Health Services Administration, 2005). Substance use differs among those who entered the military, worked, or attended college after high school, according to analyses of data from the Monitoring the Future panel, which followed high school seniors 1 and 2 years after graduation and subsequently at 2-year intervals. Those who entered the military were 2.5 times more likely to smoke half a pack a day 1–2 years after graduation compared with those who entered college; rates of heavy drinking and illicit drug use were similar among these two groups 1–2 years after graduation. Further, rates of illicit drug use declined among both recruits and civilians, but declined more among military recruits after joining the military than among civilians. Thus, military substance abuse policy may deter illicit drug use among recruits and discourage some smokers from entering the military (Bachman, Freedman-Doan, O'Malley, Johnston, & Segal, 1999).

3.2 Trends in Substance Use and Related Consequences in the Military

Similar to trends in the U.S. civilian population, active duty military personnel have seen long-term declines in cigarette use, dramatic declines in illicit drug use accompanied by recent increases, and relative stability in heavy alcohol use, along with recent increases. Figure 3.1 presents these long-term substance use trends from 1980 to 2008 (the most recent year for which data are available using the same methodology and measures) based on findings from the DoD Survey of Health Related Behaviors Among Active Duty Military Personnel (HRB survey) (Bray, Pemberton et al., 2009; Bray et al., 2010). For the HRB survey, illicit drug use in the past month is defined as use of marijuana or hashish, cocaine (including crack), hallucinogens, heroin, methamphetamine, inhalants, and GHB/GBL as well as the nonmedical use of prescription-type amphetamines/stimulants, tranquilizers/muscle relaxers, barbiturates/sedatives, and pain relievers. Heavy alcohol use is defined as drinking five or more drinks per typical drinking occasion at least once a week in the 30 days before the survey. Past month cigarette use is defined as having smoked at least 100 cigarettes in one's lifetime and having smoked a cigarette in the past 30 days. More complete definitions of these variables are included in Chap. 2. Among all active duty military personnel, past month cigarette use declined significantly from 51.0 % in 1980 to 30.6 % in 2008, with significant decreases between most survey years. Heavy cigarette use (smoking a pack or more of cigarettes per day) also decreased between 1980 and 2008, from 34.2 % to 10.0 %. Smokeless tobacco use (the use of products such as chewing tobacco or snuff) was more stable during the period for which information on use was available: 13.2 % of military personnel used smokeless tobacco in 1995 and 13.6 % did so in 2008. Data for heavy cigarette use and smokeless tobacco use are not presented in Fig. 3.1.

The rate of illicit drug use was high in 1980—27.6 % of military personnel used an illicit drug in the past month—but this rate declined dramatically through the

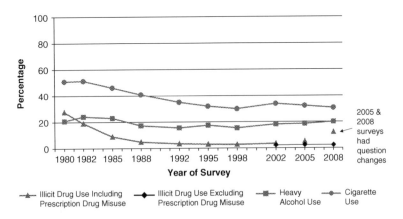

Fig. 3.1 Trends in substance use in the past month among DoD personnel, 1980–2008

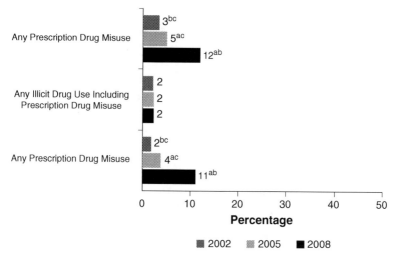

Fig. 3.2 Trends in categories of illicit drug use in the past month among DoD personnel, 2002–2008
[a]Estimate is significantly significant from the 2002 estimate at the .05 level
[b]Estimate is significantly significant from the 2005 estimate at the .05 level
[c]Estimate is significantly significant from the 2008 estimate at the .05 level

1980s and 1990s. Between 1992 and 2002, about 3 % of military personnel used illicit drugs in the past month. In 2005 and 2008, questionnaire changes in the HRB survey rendered the findings on illicit drug use not directly comparable to prior years. In the 2005 HRB survey, examples of specific types of illicit drugs were added for clarity; in 2008, questions about illegal drugs and prescription drugs were asked separately, and questions about "analgesics" were changed to "pain relievers." The set of questions about prescription drug misuse, or nonmedical use of these drugs, asked whether these drugs were taken without a doctor's prescription, in greater amounts or more often than prescribed, or for reasons such as to get "high" or for "thrills" or "kicks." Use of over-the-counter drugs was excluded. Changes in questionnaire wording are described in more detail in Chap. 2. The result may have been an increase in the measured prevalence of illicit drugs overall in 2005 and 2008 and in the use of specific classes of illicit drugs, notably, prescription drugs used for nonmedical purposes.

The rate of past month illicit drug use increased from 5.0 % in 2005 to 12.0 % in 2008, suggesting an increase in illicit drug use over the past decade. However, excluding prescription drug misuse, 2.2 % of military personnel reported past month illicit drug use in 2005, and 2.3 % did so in 2008, indicating that the increase in overall illicit drug use from 2005 to 2008 was largely due to an increase in prescription drug misuse. The rate of prescription drug misuse was 3.8 % in 2005 and 11.1 % in 2008. This increase was largely driven by an increase in misuse of prescription pain relievers. Bray et al. (2012) suggest that the increase in misuse of pain medications may be related to the availability of these drugs by prescription and their use in chronic pain management related to high rates of injury among military personnel.

Changes in illicit drug use between 2002 and 2008 are shown more directly in the categories of drug use presented in Fig. 3.2. As shown, use of illicit drugs

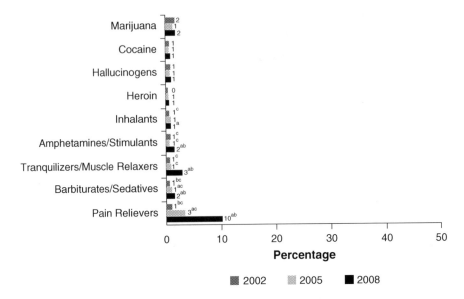

Fig. 3.3 Trends in use of selected illicit drugs in the past month among DoD personnel, 2002–2008
[a]Estimate is statistically significant from the 2002 estimate at the .05 level
[b]Estimate is statistically significant from the 2005 estimate at the .05 level
[c]Estimate is statistically significant from the 2008 estimate at the .05 level

excluding prescription drug misuse was stable at 2 % between 2002 and 2008, while use of illicit drugs including prescription drug misuse increased from 3 to 12 %, largely due to the increases in prescription drug misuse from 2 to 11 % during the same time period. These changes contrast with the stability of past month illicit drug use among the civilian adult population aged 18 and older between 2002 and 2008 at 7.9 % and the stability of nonmedical use of prescription-type drugs at 2.5 % (Substance Abuse and Mental Health Services Administration, 2011a). However, findings may differ for different age groups in the civilian population.

Information on the use of specific illicit drugs and classes of drugs is shown in Fig. 3.3; estimates are rounded to the nearest whole number. Note that the cocaine estimate includes crack cocaine, and the estimate for amphetamines/stimulants includes methamphetamine. For all of these specific drugs and classes of drugs, the highest prevalence of use was for pain relievers. Misuse of pain relievers increased significantly in 2002, 2005, and 2008. In contrast to illicit drug use among the adult civilian population, among whom marijuana was the most commonly used drug in 2010 (Substance Abuse and Mental Health Services Administration, 2011a), pain reliever misuse was the most common form of illicit drug use among military personnel. Significant increases were found in misuse of four types of prescription medications between 2002 and 2008, but rates of use of the other types of drugs were more stable; only inhalant use increased significantly from 2002 to 2008.

Returning to Fig. 3.1, heavy alcohol use decreased between 1980 and 1988, showed some fluctuations between 1988 and 1998, increased significantly from 1998 to 2002, and continued to increase gradually in 2005 and 2008. The heavy

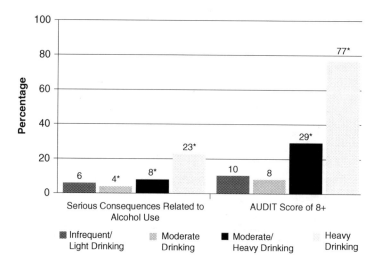

Fig. 3.4 Serious consequences related to alcohol use and alcohol dependence symptoms by drinking level, 2008
*Estimate is statistically significant from the Infrequent/Light Drinking estimate at the .05 level

drinking rate for 2008 did not differ significantly from when the survey series began in 1980. Of note, however, heavy alcohol use showed a gradual and significant increase during the decade from 1998 to 2008 (from 15 to 20 %). At the same time, there was a significant increase in the percentage of alcohol abstainers among military personnel, from 13.5 % in 1980 to 21.6 % in 2008 (data not shown in Fig. 3.1) indicating that overall rates of alcohol use have been declining, even though rates of heavy use have not. Similar to the upward trend in heavy drinking from 1998 to 2008, binge drinking (five or more drinks per occasion at least once in the past month) also showed a steady increase during this decade from 35 to 47 % (data not shown in Fig. 3.1) (Bray, Brown, & Williams, 2013).

Heavy and binge drinking among military personnel is a persistent problem related to military culture that supports and facilitates excessive alcohol use (Ames & Cunradi, 2006). Heavy drinking among military personnel is of particular concern because heavy drinking is related to engaging in other high-risk behaviors such as not wearing seatbelts, driving considerably over the speed limit, and smoking more than a pack of cigarettes a day (Williams, Bell, & Amoroso, 2002). New onset heavy drinking, binge drinking, and alcohol-related problems were found among service members with combat exposure (Jacobson et al., 2008).

The relationship between varied levels of drinking and adverse consequences and risk for alcohol problems associated with drinking is shown in Fig. 3.4. Serious consequences related to alcohol use and risk for alcohol-related problems based on the Alcohol Use Disorders Identification Test (AUDIT) defined in Chap. 2, are substantially greater among military personnel who were heavy drinkers than those who drank at lower quantities and frequencies. Almost one-fourth of heavy drinkers had experienced serious consequences related to alcohol use, and about

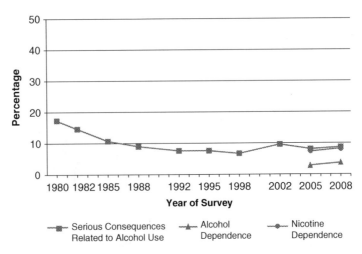

Fig. 3.5 Trends in consequences of substance use in the past year among DoD personnel, 1980–2008

three-fourths were considered at risk for alcohol problems (see also Mattiko, Rae Olmsted, Brown, & Bray, 2011).

Declines in cigarette smoking among military personnel mirror long-term trends found in the civilian population related to increasing awareness of the health risks of smoking but also reflect increasing restrictions placed on smoking in the military and the civilian sector. The dramatic decreases in illicit drug use over the period are a reflection of the stringent military policies against drug use beginning in the 1970s and 1980s, while the recent observed increases in illicit drug use may be partially related to measurement changes in the HRB survey but also to increases in prescription drug misuse in both the military and civilian sectors (U.S. Department of the Army, 2012). Increases in prescription drug misuse among military personnel may also be related to the availability of pain medications prescribed to control chronic pain related to injury. Indeed, the most important predictor of prescription pain medication misuse in the military is having a prescription for pain medication (Bray et al., 2012).

Trends in serious consequences related to alcohol use among military personnel show a long-term decline from 1980 to 1998, followed by recent increases, as shown in Fig. 3.5. As defined in Chap. 2, the measure of serious consequences related to alcohol use includes experiencing one or more problems related to alcohol use, including being passed over for a promotion, losing a week or more from work, and alcohol-related accident or arrest other than driving under the influence. Based on data from the HRB survey, 17.3 % of military personnel reported serious alcohol-related consequences in the past year in 1980, but only 8.7 % did so in 2008. Data on alcohol dependence using a score of 20 or higher on the AUDIT (see Chap. 2) are available only for 2005 and 2008. These data show that 2.9 % of military personnel exhibited alcohol dependence in 2005 and 3.8 % did so in 2008, a change that was not statistically significant. Similarly, according to NSDUH, alcohol dependence and abuse were stable among civilian adults between 2009 and 2010, but showed a small but significant decline between 2005 and 2010 (Substance Abuse and Mental Health Services Administration, 2011a). Although the measures used in NSDUH and the HRB surveys are not directly comparable (NSDUH reports measures of alcohol dependence or abuse and the HRB survey reports measures of alcohol dependence), the trends in these measures are similar. Nicotine dependence was evident among 7.6 % of military personnel in 2005 and 8.3 % in 2008, which is a nonsignificant difference (measures of nicotine dependence were not available for other years). These rates were nearly identical to those for serious consequences for those years.

Although heavy alcohol use has been relatively stable among military personnel, serious consequences from alcohol use have decreased suggesting that personnel drinking at other (non-heavy) levels also were at risk for consequences. The decreases in serious consequences may be related to the military placing increasing restrictions on alcohol use, including banning happy hours and placing a greater focus on responsible drinking.

3.3 Military and Civilian Comparisons

To help gauge the progress of military policies and programs, the military often looks to civilian data. Rates of substance use in 2008 among military personnel and civilians were examined by comparing data for military personnel from the 2008 HRB survey and for civilians from the 2007 NSDUH. Data were considered for those aged 18–64 in both populations and for only the U.S.-based military personnel (including Alaska and Hawaii). To further increase comparability of the two datasets, civilian data were standardized to the sociodemographic distribution of the U.S.-based military population by gender, age, education, and marital status. These adjustments were made to enable comparison of substance use in the two populations, which differ in sociodemographic characteristics related to variation in rates of substance use. The civilian estimates were recalculated using the adjusted demographics. Overall, comparisons revealed that the rate of illicit drug use was lower among military personnel than among civilians, rates of binge drinking and heavy drinking were higher among military personnel than among civilians, and the rate of cigarette smoking was similar between the two populations (Fig. 3.6).

Rates of past month illicit drug use, including and excluding the misuse of prescription drugs, were lower among military personnel than among civilians in 2008, although misuse of prescription drugs alone was higher among military personnel than among civilians. Among individuals aged 18–64, the rate of past month use of illicit drugs including prescription drugs was lower among military personnel than among civilians: at 12.6 and 14.2 %, respectively. Similarly, the rate of illicit drug use excluding prescription drugs was lower among military personnel than among civilians: 2.3 and 12.0 %, respectively. However, for prescription drug misuse alone,

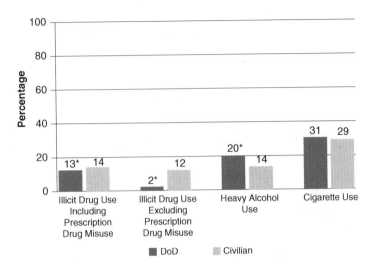

Fig. 3.6 Standardized comparisons of substance use in the past month among DoD personnel and civilians aged 18–64, 2008
*Estimate is statistically significant from the Civilian estimate at the .05 level
Source: Civilian data are from 2007 National Survey on Drug Use and Health

military personnel were more likely than civilians to misuse these drugs: 11.7 % of military personnel and 4.4 % of civilians.

Some differences in the findings of the lower overall rates of illicit drug use among military personnel compared with civilians were found by gender and age group among persons aged 18–64. Similar to findings for all persons aged 18–64, rates were lower for military personnel than civilians for any illicit drug including prescription drug misuse for males and for persons aged 18–25 and for any illicit drug excluding prescription drug misuse for males and females and all age groups. In contrast, use was greater among military personnel than civilians for use of any illicit drug including prescription drug misuse for females and for persons aged 35–64 and for prescription drug misuse among males and females and for all age groups. These comparisons by age group are shown in Fig. 3.7. These findings appear to be driven by the consistently higher rates of misuse of prescription drugs among all groups of military personnel compared to civilians.

In 2008, rates of heavy drinking and binge drinking were higher among military personnel than among civilians for both males and females and for most age groups. For example, 19.7 % of military personnel aged 18–64 were heavy drinkers compared with 13.6 % of civilians in that age range. Rates of heavy drinking were greater among military personnel than civilians who were aged 18–35, similar among military personnel and civilians who were aged 36–45, and lower among military personnel than civilians who were aged 46–64. Comparisons for heavy alcohol use by age group are shown in Fig. 3.8.

Comparisons for binge drinking among military and civilians are similar to those for heavy drinking; only binge drinkers had much higher rates. More than four in ten military personnel and civilians were binge drinkers. Military personnel (45.8 %)

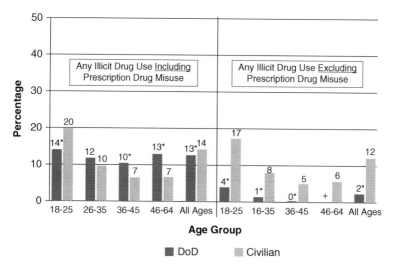

Fig. 3.7 Standardized comparisons of any illicit drug use in the past month among DoD personnel and civilians by age group, 2008
*Estimate is statistically significant from the Civilian estimate at the .05 level
+Estimate is suppressed
Source: Civilian data are from 2007 National Survey on Drug Use and Health

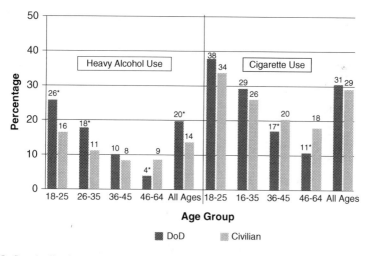

Fig. 3.8 Standardized comparisons of heavy alcohol use and cigarette use in the past month among DoD personnel and civilians by age group, 2008
*Estimate is statistically significant from the Civilian estimate at the .05 level
Source: Civilian data are from 2007 National Survey on Drug Use and Health

were more likely than civilians (40.6 %) to be binge drinkers. These finding were also related to age. Rates of binge drinking were greater among military personnel than civilians for younger persons, but among older persons rates of binge drinking were lower among military personnel or similar between the two populations.

Overall rates of cigarette smoking among military personnel and civilians in 2008 were similar: 30.5 % of military personnel and 29.1 % of civilians aged 18–64 smoked cigarettes in the past month. These findings held for both males and females, although the rates of smoking differed for older age groups. As shown in Fig. 3.8, among persons aged 36–45 and 46–64, cigarette smoking was more common among civilians than among military personnel, but cigarette smoking was similar among military personnel and civilians in the younger age groups.

Other factors being equal, rates of substance use among military personnel and civilians should be similar because military personnel are drawn from the civilian population, and these analyses controlled for some differences in the sociodemographic composition of the two populations that could account for some variation in rates. Remaining differences could be associated with specific conditions in military or civilian life. The overall lower rates of illicit drug use among military personnel than among civilians are likely a reflection of the stringent military policies against drug use, and the higher rates of heavy alcohol use are likely related to a military culture that facilitates heavy drinking (Ames & Cunradi, 2006; Institute of Medicine [IOM], 2012). Rates of cigarette smoking are similar among military personnel and civilians, and declining in both populations, indicating the presence of stringent anti-smoking policies in both military and civilian environments. However, differentials for specific drugs or by gender or age group suggest differences in substance use between military and civilian populations. Although illicit drug use is generally lower among military personnel than civilians, prescription drug misuse is consistently higher among military personnel compared with civilians. Rates of heavy drinking and binge drinking were higher for younger military personnel than younger civilians, while rates were more similar for older persons. In contrast, the rate of cigarette smoking was lower among older military personnel than civilians but more similar among younger persons. These findings suggest that some of the higher rates of use of some substances for younger military personnel than younger civilians may diminish as military personnel age.

3.4 Correlates and Predictors of Substance Use and Abuse

In 2008, 12.0 % of active duty military personnel used illicit drugs including prescription drugs in the past month, 20.0 % were heavy drinkers, and 30.6 % smoked cigarettes in the past month, as shown in Table 3.1. Some similarities and differences in the prevalence of substance use were seen across sociodemographic characteristics for the three measures. Rates of illicit drug use, heavy drinking, and cigarette smoking were all higher among less educated persons than more highly educated persons and among younger persons than older persons. Illicit drug use was greater among females than males, while heavy drinking and cigarette smoking were greater among males than females. Illicit drug use was higher among African Americans than white non-Hispanics; heavy drinking was higher among whites and Hispanics than other racial/ethnic groups; and cigarette smoking was higher among whites than other racial/ethnic groups.

Table 3.1 Illicit drug use, heavy alcohol use, and cigarette use in the past month, by selected sociodemographic characteristics, 2008

Sociodemographic characteristic	Illicit drug use	Heavy alcohol use	Cigarette use
Gender			
Male	11.8 (0.4)	22.0 (1.2)	32.3 (1.2)
Female	13.4 (0.6)	8.3 (0.6)	20.8 (1.5)
Age			
20 or younger	13.6 (0.7)	19.1 (1.7)	36.8 (2.6)
21–25	13.1 (0.6)	29.6 (1.6)	38.1 (1.3)
26–34	11.3 (0.6)	18.7 (0.7)	30.5 (1.1)
35 or older	10.4 (0.7)	9.6 (0.5)	17.0 (1.0)
Race/ethnicity			
White non-Hispanic	10.7 (0.5)	21.5 (1.1)	34.3 (1.4)
African American non-Hispanic	15.4 (0.9)	13.8 (1.2)	19.7 (1.2)
Hispanic	14.2 (1.0)	22.9 (1.7)	27.0 (1.2)
Other	12.4 (0.8)	16.8 (1.2)	28.6 (1.5)
Education			
High school or less	14.7 (0.7)	27.8 (1.7)	43.0 (1.7)
Some college	12.2 (0.4)	19.8 (0.9)	31.6 (1.0)
College graduate or higher	7.7 (0.5)	9.5 (0.6)	10.9 (0.6)
Family status			
Not married	13.1 (0.6)	25.6 (1.6)	35.1 (1.4)
Married, spouse not present	14.3 (1.0)	20.8 (1.6)	31.2 (1.6)
Married, spouse present	10.5 (0.4)	14.4 (0.8)	26.3 (1.3)
Pay grade			
E1–E3	14.5 (0.7)	24.9 (1.9)	39.6 (2.9)
E4–E6	13.1 (0.6)	23.2 (1.2)	36.3 (0.8)
E7–E9	11.5 (1.1)	12.9 (0.7)	20.5 (1.3)
W1–W5	6.4 (2.2)	16.8 (1.6)	14.6 (1.0)
O1–O3	5.2 (0.5)	10.7 (0.6)	10.1 (0.7)
O4–O10	7.0 (1.2)	5.0 (0.8)	5.5 (1.2)
Total	12.0 (0.4)	20.0 (1.1)	30.6 (1.2)

Source: DoD Survey of Health Related Behaviors among Active Duty Military Personnel, 2008
Note: Table displays the percentages of military personnel in each sociodemographic group that reported substance use in the past month. The standard error of each estimate is presented in parentheses.

The predictors of substance use and abuse are examined more closely in the results of regression models for the following six outcome measures: illicit drug use in the past month (including prescription drug misuse), heavy drinking, cigarette smoking in the past month, serious alcohol consequences, alcohol dependence, and nicotine dependence. Following the conceptual framework presented in Chap. 1, regression models were developed for each outcome measure, with predictors including sociodemographic characteristics (gender, age, race/ethnicity, family status, presence of children), military conditions (pay grade, branch of the services, deployment and combat exposure, region where stationed), and psychosocial characteristics (history of physical or sexual abuse, risk-taking or impulsivity, spirituality, and active coping). Each model also included other key outcome measures as predictors: substance use, health status and health behaviors, and mental health problems. These variables are all defined in Chap. 2. Overall, these predictors account for between 5 and 18 % of the variance in each of the six outcome measures.

Table 3.2 presents findings of the regression models for illicit drug use, heavy alcohol use, and cigarette use.

3.4.1   Illicit Drug Use

In 2008, significant predictors of illicit drug use in the past month were gender, race/ethnicity, pay grade, service, deployment and combat exposure, risk-taking, illness, injury, heavy drinking, smoking, and screening positive for posttraumatic stress disorder (PTSD). Controlling for other variables, illicit drug use was higher among women than men; among whites compared with African Americans; among those in pay grades E1–E3 compared with senior officers; among those with moderate combat exposure compared with those who had not been deployed; and among risk-takers, those who had experienced illness or injury in the past 12 months, heavy drinkers, smokers, and those who had screened positive for PTSD compared with others who did not possess these characteristics. Screening positive for PTSD, heavy drinking, illness, injury, risk-taking, and junior pay grade were among the stronger predictors of illicit drug use. Those screening positive for PTSD were 1.75 times more likely than those not screening positive for PTSD to have used illicit drugs in the past month. Pay grades E1–E3 were 1.64 times more likely than pay grades O4–O10 to have used illicit drugs in the past month. Similarly, heavy drinkers were 1.63 times more likely than those who were not heavy drinkers to have used illicit drugs in the past month. Illicit drug use was unrelated to age group, family status, presence of children in the home, region where stationed, history of physical/sexual abuse, spirituality, exercise, screening positive for depression, screening positive for anxiety, high work or family stress, or active coping.

3.4.2   Heavy Drinking

Gender, age group, race/ethnicity, family status, presence of children, pay grade, deployment and combat exposure, risk-taking, spirituality, illicit drug use, smoking, screening positive for PTSD, and high work or family stress in the past 12 months were significant predictors of heavy drinking. Heavy drinking was greater among males than females, persons aged 21–25 and 26–34 compared with those aged 35 and older, whites and Hispanics compared with African Americans, persons with children not living with them, personnel in the Marine Corps compared with those in the Air Force, those deployed and with a high level of combat exposure, risk-takers, illicit drug users, smokers, and those who indicated high work or family stress. Gender, cigarette smoking, and age were among the strongest predictors of heavy drinking. Men were 2.78 times more likely than women to be heavy drinkers,

Table 3.2 Correlates of illicit drug use, heavy alcohol use, and cigarette use in past month, 2008

Independent variables	Illicit drug use			Heavy alcohol use			Cigarette use		
	Unadjusted %	Adjusted %	Adjusted ORs[a] (95 % CI)[b]	Unadjusted %	Adjusted %	Adjusted ORs[a] (95 % CI)[b]	Unadjusted %	Adjusted %	Adjusted ORs[a] (95 % CI)[b]
Gender									
Male	11.8	8.8	1.00	22.0	16.9	1.00	32.3	26.3	1.00
Female	13.4	10.7	1.24* (1.09–1.41)	8.3	6.8	0.36* (0.30–0.44)	20.8	19.4	0.67* (0.58–0.78)
Age									
20 or younger	13.6	9.0	0.95 (0.70–1.28)	19.1	10.3	0.95 (0.64–1.41)	36.8	24.7	1.18 (0.91–1.54)
21–25	13.1	8.9	0.94 (0.78–1.15)	29.6	21.0	2.20* (1.73–2.80)	38.1	26.9	1.32* (1.10–1.60)
26–34	11.3	9.0	0.95 (0.77–1.17)	18.7	15.8	1.56* (1.34–1.81)	30.5	26.7	1.31* (1.12–1.53)
35 or older	10.4	9.4	1.00	9.6	10.8	1.00	17.0	21.8	1.00
Race/ethnicity									
White non-Hispanic	10.7	8.2	0.66* (0.54–0.80)	21.5	15.4	1.23* (1.07–1.41)	34.3	28.9	2.13* (1.88–2.40)
African American non-Hispanic	15.4	12.0	1.00	13.8	12.9	1.00	19.7	16.1	1.00
Hispanic	14.2	10.2	0.84 (0.63–1.11)	22.9	17.2	1.40* (1.16–1.70)	27.0	18.7	1.20* (1.04–1.40)
Other	12.4	10.5	0.87 (0.65–1.15)	16.8	12.3	0.95 (0.79–1.14)	28.6	24.8	1.72* (1.48–2.01)
Family status									
Not married	13.1	9.4	1.10 (0.90–1.34)	25.6	17.8	1.56* (1.32–1.83)	35.1	25.7	1.07 (0.95–1.21)
Married–spouse not present	14.3	10.1	1.18 (0.93–1.51)	20.8	16.5	1.41* (1.17–1.71)	31.2	27.2	1.16 (0.95–1.42)
Married–spouse present	10.5	8.6	1.00	14.4	12.2	1.00	26.4	24.4	1.00
Children living with you									
Yes	11.4	9.4	1.07 (0.88–1.31)	13.8	13.0	0.78* (0.70–0.86)	26.3	26.8	1.15* (1.04–1.27)
No	12.3	8.9	1.00	24.0	16.2	1.00	33.4	24.1	1.00

(continued)

Table 3.2 (continued)

Independent variables	Illicit drug use			Heavy alcohol use			Cigarette use		
	Unadjusted %	Adjusted %	Adjusted ORs[a] (95 % CI)[b]	Unadjusted %	Adjusted %	Adjusted ORs[a] (95 % CI)[b]	Unadjusted %	Adjusted %	Adjusted ORs[a] (95 % CI)[b]
Pay grade									
E1–E3	14.5	11.5	1.64* (1.04–2.59)	24.9	17.1	1.80* (1.08–3.01)	39.6	38.0	9.38* (5.95–14.79)
E4–E6	13.2	9.6	1.35 (0.92–1.98)	23.2	15.0	1.54* (1.01–2.35)	36.3	31.3	6.97* (4.80–10.11)
E7–E9	11.5	9.3	1.30 (0.96–1.76)	12.9	16.9	1.78* (1.15–2.75)	20.5	21.6	4.23* (2.78–6.42)
W1–W5	6.4	5.8	0.78 (0.29–2.07)	16.8	18.2	1.94* (1.29–2.90)	14.6	10.2	1.74* (1.04–2.91)
O1–O3	5.2	5.3	0.71 (0.40–1.24)	10.7	11.3	1.11 (0.70–1.76)	10.1	9.9	1.68* (1.12–2.52)
O4–O10	7.0	7.3	1.00	5.0	10.3	1.00	5.5	6.1	1.00
Service									
Army	15.8	11.3	1.58* (1.29–1.94)	21.8	14.8	1.08 (0.83–1.41)	33.3	27.9	1.52* (1.23–1.88)
Navy	10.2	8.4	1.14 (0.94–1.39)	18.0	13.9	1.01 (0.86–1.18)	30.7	26.0	1.38* (1.18–1.62)
Marine Corps	12.1	8.1	1.09 (0.92–1.28)	29.3	18.9	1.45* (1.21–1.74)	37.4	26.2	1.39* (1.15–1.70)
Air Force	7.5	7.5	1.00	14.0	13.9	1.00	22.6	20.3	1.00
Deployment and combat exposure									
Not deployed	11.2	8.4	1.00 (0.84–1.19)	18.0	13.0	0.86 (0.69–1.07)	28.3	21.5	0.80* (0.70–0.91)
Deployed-none	8.6	8.4	1.00	17.2	14.7	1.00	27.3	25.5	1.00
Deployed-moderate	10.4	9.7	1.17* (1.01–1.37)	16.3	14.2	0.96 (0.80–1.15)	28.4	27.8	1.13* (1.04–1.22)
Deployed-high	16.5	10.1	1.21 (0.95–1.55)	26.8	18.4	1.31* (1.07–1.61)	35.3	27.4	1.10 (0.97–1.25)
Region									
CONUS	12.2	9.3	1.00	19.6	14.5	1.00	29.9	24.0	1.00
OCONUS/Afloats	11.6	8.6	0.92 (0.78–1.08)	20.9	15.6	1.09 (0.94–1.28)	32.0	27.5	1.20* (1.04–1.38)
High work or family stress									
Yes	14.9	9.1	1.00 (0.91–1.11)	24.0	15.9	1.13* (1.01–1.27)	36.9	26.9	1.15* (1.04–1.28)
No	10.3	9.1	1.00	17.5	14.3	1.00	26.7	24.2	1.00

History of physical/sexual abuse								
Yes	13.8	9.0	0.98 (0.83–1.15)	22.3	15.1	1.04 (0.95–1.14)	36.6	29.9	1.51* (1.35–1.69)
No	10.5	9.2	1.00	17.8	14.6	1.00	25.5	22.0	1.00
Risk-taking/impulsivity								
Yes	21.6	11.9	1.39* (1.22–1.58)	39.9	21.0	1.59* (1.33–1.89)	48.8	29.9	1.29* (1.10–1.52)
No	11.1	8.9	1.00	18.1	14.4	1.00	28.8	24.8	1.00
Spirituality								
High	11.2	9.5	1.00	11.3	11.4	1.00	17.8	18.4	1.00
Medium	12.7	9.5	1.00 (0.82–1.21)	19.4	15.1	1.39* (1.19–1.62)	31.1	26.8	1.62* (1.45–1.81)
Low	10.9	8.0	0.83 (0.66–1.05)	26.6	17.9	1.70* (1.49–1.94)	38.0	28.8	1.79* (1.54–2.09)
Moderate/vigorous physical exercise								
Yes	12.0	9.1	1.03 (0.87–1.23)	20.1	15.0	1.11 (0.95–1.30)	29.9	24.4	0.76* (0.66–0.87)
No	12.1	8.9	1.00	19.1	13.7	1.00	33.6	29.8	1.00
Illness in past 12 months								
Yes	20.3	12.1	1.44* (1.20–1.73)	23.4	15.2	1.03 (0.84–1.28)	34.8	25.8	1.04 (0.87–1.23)
No	10.7	8.7	1.00	19.5	14.8	1.00	29.9	25.1	1.00
Injury in past 12 months								
Yes	15.3	10.6	1.39* (1.22–1.58)	21.5	15.3	1.07 (0.96–1.18)	33.3	25.9	1.07 (0.98–1.17)
No	8.8	7.8	1.00	18.6	14.4	1.00	28.0	24.5	1.00
Need for further depression evaluation								
Yes	18.7	10.6	1.24 (0.99–1.56)	27.0	14.5	0.97 (0.84–1.12)	41.3	27.5	1.16* (1.02–1.32)
No	9.8	8.7	1.00	17.7	14.9	1.00	27.3	24.6	1.00
Presence of anxiety								
Yes	20.7	9.3	1.03 (0.80–1.31)	29.0	15.9	1.10 (0.95–1.27)	42.3	26.3	1.07 (0.92–1.24)
No	10.4	9.1	1.00	18.2	14.7	1.00	28.2	25.0	1.00
Screened positive for PTSD								
Yes	25.9	14.2	1.75* (1.49–2.06)	35.5	19.8	1.47* (1.19–1.81)	46.5	25.8	1.04 (0.87–1.24)
No	10.2	8.6	1.00	17.9	14.4	1.00	28.1	25.1	1.00

(continued)

Table 3.2 (continued)

	Illicit drug use			Heavy alcohol use			Cigarette use		
Independent variables	Unadjusted %	Adjusted %	Adjusted ORs[a] (95 % CI)[b]	Unadjusted %	Adjusted %	Adjusted ORs[a] (95 % CI)[b]	Unadjusted %	Adjusted %	Adjusted ORs[a] (95 % CI)[b]
Illicit drug use in past month									
Yes	–	–	–	32.0	21.1	1.62* (1.37–1.91)	40.1	29.2	1.26* (1.05–1.50)
No	–	–	–	18.4	14.2	1.00	29.2	24.7	1.00
Heavy alcohol use in past month									
Yes	18.3	12.9	1.63* (1.39–1.92)	–	–	–	55.5	41.5	2.52* (2.28–2.79)
No	9.7	8.3	1.00	–	–	–	24.5	22.0	1.00
Cigarette use in past month									
Yes	15.8	10.5	1.26* (1.06–1.50)	36.1	25.1	2.54* (2.30–2.80)	–	–	–
No	10.3	8.5	1.00	12.8	11.7	1.00	–	–	–
Active coping	–	–	0.94 (0.86–1.04)	–	–	0.93 (0.85–1.01)	–	–	0.99 (0.90–1.07)
Total	12.0	12.0	–	20.0	20.0	–	30.6	30.6	–
R²	–	–	0.05	–	–	0.13	–	–	0.17

Source: DoD Survey of Health Related Behaviors among Active Duty Military Personnel, 2008

Note: Estimates are percentages of military personnel in each sociodemographic group that reported substance use in the past month.

*Odds ratio is significantly different from the reference group

[a]OR=Odds ratios were adjusted for all other independent variables in the model

[b]95 % CI=95 % confidence interval of the odds ratio

smokers were 2.54 times more likely than nonsmokers to be heavy drinkers, and persons aged 21–25 were 2.20 times more likely than persons aged 35 or older to be heavy drinkers. Heavy drinking was not related to region where stationed, having a history of physical or sexual abuse, exercise, illness, injury, screening positive for depression, screening positive for anxiety, or active coping.

3.4.3 Cigarette Smoking

Significant predictors of cigarette smoking in the past month were gender, age group, race/ethnicity, presence of children, pay grade, service, deployment or combat exposure, region where stationed, history of physical/sexual abuse, risk-taking, spirituality, exercise, illicit drug use, heavy drinking, screening positive for depression, and high work or family stress. Cigarette smoking was more likely among males than females, persons aged 21–34 compared with those aged 35 and older, racial/ethnic groups other than African Americans, those with children present, those in pay grades other than O4–O10, those with moderate combat exposure compared with those who had not been deployed, persons stationed in OCONUS, those with a history of physical or sexual abuse, those with medium or low spirituality, persons who did not exercise moderately or vigorously, illicit drug users, heavy drinkers, those who screened positive for depression, those with high work or family stress, and those serving in service branches other than the Air Force. Family status, illness, injury, screening positive for PTSD, and active coping were not related to cigarette smoking. Pay grade and heavy drinking were the strongest predictors of cigarette smoking. Personnel in pay grades E1–E3 were 9.38 times more likely, those in pay grades E4–E6 were 6.97 times more likely, and those in pay grades E7–E9 were 4.23 times more likely to smoke cigarettes compared with those in pay grades O4–O10. Heavy drinkers were 2.52 times more likely to smoke than non-heavy drinkers.

Each of the three measures of substance use—illicit drug use, heavy drinking, and cigarette smoking—was strongly related to other measures of substance use as well as to gender, race/ethnicity, pay grade, service, deployment and combat exposure, and risk-taking. Although illicit drug use was greater among females than males, heavy drinking and smoking were greater among males than females. Whites had lower rates of illicit drug use but higher rates of heavy drinking and smoking compared with African Americans. All three substance use measures were more common among junior enlisted personnel than among senior officers. Other predictors were not consistently related to the three measures. Active coping was not significantly related to these three substance use measures, although it was negatively related to alcohol dependence and nicotine dependence, as discussed in the following section. All three measures of substance use were significantly related to moderate or high combat exposure, indicating the toll of deployment and combat exposure on service members.

Table 3.3 presents findings of the regression models for alcohol-related serious consequences, alcohol dependence, and nicotine dependence.

Table 3.3 Correlates of serious consequences related to alcohol use, alcohol dependence, and nicotine dependence in the past year, 2008

Independent variables	Alcohol consequences			Alcohol dependence			Nicotine dependence		
	Unadjusted %	Adjusted %	Adjusted ORs[a] (95 % CI)[b]	Unadjusted %	Adjusted %	Adjusted ORs[a] (95 % CI)[b]	Unadjusted %	Adjusted %	Adjusted ORs[a] (95 % CI)[b]
Gender									
Male	9.3	4.3	1.00	5.1	1.2	1.00	9.0	1.4	1.00
Female	5.1	2.6	0.59* (0.46–0.76)	2.1	0.7	0.58* (0.41–0.83)	4.2	1.1	0.75* (0.60–0.94)
Age									
20 or younger	13.8	4.6	2.04* (1.42–2.95)	9.6	1.3	1.52 (0.76–3.05)	11.1	1.3	0.84 (0.58–1.22)
21–25	13.3	5.7	2.53* (1.83–3.50)	6.7	1.4	1.59 (1.00–2.53)	10.7	1.4	0.88 (0.68–1.14)
26–34	6.4	4.0	1.75* (1.25–2.45)	3.4	1.2	1.39 (0.88–2.20)	7.5	1.3	0.87 (0.68–1.12)
35 or older	2.4	2.3	1.00	1.3	0.9	1.00	4.2	1.5	1.00
Race/ethnicity									
White non-Hispanic	8.7	3.7	0.86 (0.70–1.06)	5.0	1.2	1.17 (0.76–1.81)	10.4	1.8	2.76* (2.01–3.78)
African American non-Hispanic	7.5	4.3	1.00	3.3	1.0	1.00	3.3	0.7	1.00
Hispanic	11.4	5.4	1.27 (0.99–1.62)	5.9	1.5	1.49* (1.03–2.16)	5.2	0.9	1.44 (0.91–2.28)
Other	8.4	3.6	0.82 (0.62–1.09)	3.7	0.9	0.90 (0.52–1.56)	6.0	1.2	1.82* (1.16–2.84)
Family status									
Not married	12.5	5.0	1.59* (1.33–1.91)	7.0	1.4	1.51* (1.03–2.21)	9.6	1.4	0.97 (0.79–1.20)
Married–spouse not present	9.4	4.2	1.33 (0.85–2.06)	6.0	1.7	1.87* (1.40–2.48)	8.4	1.6	1.18 (0.77–1.79)
Married–spouse present	4.8	3.2	1.00	2.2	0.9	1.00	7.0	1.4	1.00
Children living with you									
Yes	5.0	3.7	0.88 (0.69–1.12)	2.3	1.0	0.75 (0.48–1.18)	7.1	1.5	1.15 (0.96–1.37)
No	11.0	4.1	1.00	6.2	1.3	1.00	9.0	1.3	1.00

Pay grade									
E1–E3	15.9	5.3	1.09 (0.61–1.94)	9.7	1.5	0.66 (0.27–1.60)	12.3	1.9	2.51* (1.48–4.28)
E4–E6	9.2	4.0	0.80 (0.42–1.53)	4.8	1.0	0.45* (0.21–0.98)	9.5	1.5	1.98* (1.22–3.22)
E7–E9	2.3	2.5	0.49 (0.24–1.02)	1.1	0.8	0.36* (0.16–0.83)	4.8	1.4	1.83* (1.14–2.93)
W1–W5	4.2	4.1	0.82 (0.54–1.26)	3.7	2.3	1.04 (0.29–3.71)	3.7	1.1	1.47 (0.85–2.53)
O1–O3	2.4	2.9	0.59 (0.26–1.31)	1.5	1.2	0.56 (0.26–1.19)	1.6	0.7	0.87 (0.48–1.61)
O4–O10	2.0	4.9	1.00	1.3	2.2	1.00	1.4	0.8	1.00
Service									
Army	10.0	4.2	1.30 (0.98–1.74)	5.5	1.3	1.41* (1.05–1.91)	11.1	1.9	1.79* (1.37–2.35)
Navy	8.1	4.1	1.28 (0.90–1.82)	4.2	1.2	1.32 (0.91–1.91)	6.4	1.1	1.03 (0.84–1.26)
Marine Corps	14.2	4.8	1.50* (1.08–2.08)	8.3	1.1	1.19 (0.91–1.55)	10.2	1.4	1.26* (1.03–1.53)
Air Force	4.2	3.2	1.00	2.1	0.9	1.00	4.4	1.1	1.00
Deployment and combat exposure									
Not deployed	9.1	3.9	1.04 (0.82–1.33)	4.7	1.0	0.78 (0.55–1.11)	7.6	1.3	0.85 (0.66–1.10)
Deployed-none	5.8	3.8	1.00	3.0	1.3	1.00	6.3	1.6	1.00
Deployed-moderate	5.7	3.7	0.98 (0.76–1.28)	2.4	1.1	0.85 (0.58–1.26)	6.3	1.3	0.85 (0.67–1.08)
Deployed-high	11.6	4.4	1.17 (0.89–1.54)	7.4	1.3	1.01 (0.66–1.56)	11.3	1.4	0.88 (0.63–1.22)
Region									
CONUS	8.9	4.0	1.00	4.9	1.2	1.00	8.4	1.4	1.00
OCONUS/Afloats	8.4	3.9	0.98 (0.80–1.20)	4.5	1.1	0.87 (0.61–1.24)	8.0	1.4	0.97 (0.82–1.16)
High work or family stress									
Yes	12.2	4.2	1.12 (0.90–1.39)	7.2	1.4	1.35* (1.12–1.63)	11.2	1.5	1.11 (0.95–1.30)
No	6.4	3.8	1.00	3.1	1.0	1.00	6.3	1.3	1.00
History of physical/sexual abuse									
Yes	12.1	5.1	1.57* (1.29–1.90)	6.0	1.1	0.97 (0.81–1.15)	10.5	1.5	1.19* (1.04–1.35)
No	5.8	3.3	1.00	3.4	1.2	1.00	6.2	1.3	1.00
Risk-taking/impulsivity									
Yes	26.4	7.1	1.96* (1.61–2.39)	17.3	2.3	2.18* (1.75–2.71)	20.1	2.1	1.55* (1.24–1.93)
No	6.9	3.7	1.00	3.4	1.1	1.00	7.1	1.3	1.00

(continued)

Table 3.3 (continued)

Independent variables	Alcohol consequences			Alcohol dependence			Nicotine dependence		
	Unadjusted %	Adjusted %	Adjusted ORs[a] (95 % CI)[b]	Unadjusted %	Adjusted %	Adjusted ORs[a] (95 % CI)[b]	Unadjusted %	Adjusted %	Adjusted ORs[a] (95 % CI)[b]
Spirituality									
High	5.1	3.0	1.00	3.2	1.1	1.00	4.6	1.6	1.00
Medium	8.9	4.5	1.53* (1.23–1.91)	3.9	1.1	1.02 (0.78–1.34)	7.3	1.3	0.79* (0.62–0.99)
Low	10.1	3.9	1.33* (1.02–1.73)	6.2	1.3	1.19 (0.87–1.63)	11.8	1.5	0.93 (0.68–1.27)
Moderate/vigorous physical exercise									
Yes	8.5	3.9	0.87 (0.70–1.09)	4.4	1.1	0.95 (0.66–1.36)	7.7	1.3	0.81* (0.66–0.99)
No	9.0	4.4	1.00	5.9	1.2	1.00	10.2	1.7	1.00
Illness in past 12 months									
Yes	15.5	5.2	1.40* (1.11–1.78)	8.8	1.5	1.40 (0.99–1.97)	11.7	1.6	1.16 (0.96–1.41)
No	7.6	3.8	1.00	4.0	1.1	1.00	7.7	1.4	1.00
Injury in past 12 months									
Yes	10.9	4.4	1.25* (1.11–1.42)	5.4	1.1	0.85 (0.59–1.22)	9.7	1.4	1.07 (0.92–1.24)
No	6.6	3.5	1.00	4.0	1.3	1.00	6.9	1.3	1.00
Need for further depression evaluation									
Yes	16.1	4.9	1.31* (1.09–1.58)	10.4	1.6	1.57* (1.16–2.14)	13.6	1.4	0.99 (0.80–1.21)
No	6.3	3.7	1.00	2.9	1.0	1.00	6.5	1.4	1.00
Presence of anxiety									
Yes	16.9	4.0	1.00 (0.78–1.30)	12.3	1.6	1.45* (1.07–1.97)	15.8	1.8	1.32* (1.04–1.66)
No	7.0	3.9	1.00	3.3	1.1	1.00	6.7	1.3	1.00
Screened positive for PTSD									
Yes	22.0	5.1	1.33* (1.10–1.62)	16.7	2.2	2.13* (1.38–3.30)	18.7	1.8	1.34 (0.94–1.92)
No	6.8	3.8	1.00	3.0	1.1	1.00	6.7	1.4	1.00

Illicit drug use in past month									
Yes	21.2	7.3	2.08* (1.73–2.51)	13.3	2.3	2.21* (1.76–2.78)	14.9	1.9	1.44* (1.11–1.86)
No	6.9	3.7	1.00	3.4	1.1	1.00	7.3	1.3	1.00
Heavy alcohol use in past month									
Yes	22.7	8.9	2.94* (2.49–3.46)	14.2	5.1	7.63* (5.17–11.25)	17.6	1.7	1.26* (1.04–1.53)
No	4.6	3.2	1.00	1.1	0.7	1.00	5.8	1.3	1.00
Cigarette use in past month									
Yes	16.4	5.9	1.84* (1.46–2.32)	9.0	1.6	1.65* (1.29–2.12)	25.4	16.9	44.65* (19.05–104.64)
No	5.2	3.3	1.00	2.5	1.0	1.00	0.7	0.5	1.00
Active coping	–	–	1.07 (0.95–1.19)	–	–	0.83* (0.73–0.94)	–	–	0.72* (0.64–0.80)
Total	8.7	8.7	–	4.7	4.7	–	8.3	8.3	–
R^2	–	–	0.11	–	–	0.10	–	–	0.18

Source: DoD Survey of Health Related Behaviors among Active Duty Military Personnel, 2008

Note: Estimates are percentages among military personnel in each sociodemographic group.

*Odds ratio is significantly different from the reference group

[a]OR = Odds ratios were adjusted for all other independent variables in the model

[b]95 % CI = 95 % confidence interval of the odds ratio

3.4.4 Alcohol-Related Serious Consequences

Significant predictors of serious consequences related to alcohol in the past year were gender, age group, family status, service, history of physical or sexual abuse, risk-taking, spirituality, illness, injury, illicit drug use, heavy drinking, smoking, screening positive for depression, and screening positive for PTSD. Serious alcohol consequences were more likely among males than females, persons younger than age 35 compared with those aged 35 and older, unmarried persons, those in the Marine Corps compared with those in the Air Force, those with a history of physical or sexual abuse, risk-takers, those with medium or low spirituality, those with illness or injury, illicit drug users, heavy drinkers, and those who screened positive for depression or PTSD. Among the strongest predictors of serious alcohol consequences were age, illicit drug use, and heavy drinking: persons aged 25 or younger, illicit drug users, and heavy drinkers were more than twice as likely as their counterparts to experience serious consequences related to alcohol use. Serious alcohol consequences were not related to race/ethnicity, presence of children, pay grade, deployment or combat exposure, region where stationed, exercise, screening positive for anxiety, high work or family stress, and active coping.

3.4.5 Alcohol Dependence

Significant predictors of alcohol dependence were gender, race/ethnicity, family status, pay grade, service, risk-taking, illicit drug use, cigarette smoking, screening positive for depression or anxiety, screening positive for PTSD, high work or family stress, and active coping. Alcohol dependence was greater among males than females, Hispanics compared with African Americans, unmarried persons and married persons without their spouse present, persons in the Army compared with persons in the Air Force, risk-takers, illicit drug users, heavy drinkers, smokers, those screening positive for depression or anxiety, those screening positive for PTSD, those with high work or family stress, and those with less active coping skills. Alcohol dependence was lower among those in pay grades E4–E6 and E7–E9 compared with senior officers. In addition to heavy drinking, risk-taking, illicit drug use, and screening positive for PTSD were among the stronger predictors of alcohol dependence. Heavy drinkers were 7.63 times more likely to develop alcohol dependence, and alcohol dependence was more than twice as likely among those who were risk-takers, screened positive for PTSD, or used illicit drugs in the past month. Alcohol dependence was unrelated to age, presence of children, deployment or combat exposure, spirituality, illness, and injury.

3.4.6 Nicotine Dependence

Significant predictors of nicotine dependence were gender, race/ethnicity, pay grade, service, history of physical or sexual abuse, risk-taking, spirituality, exercise, illicit drug use, heavy drinking, smoking, screening positive for anxiety, and active coping skills. In addition to the strong correlation with smoking, nicotine dependence was higher among males than females, whites and Hispanics compared with African Americans, enlisted pay grades compared with senior officers, Army and Marine Corps personnel compared with Air Force personnel, those with a history of physical or sexual abuse, risk-takers, illicit drug users, heavy drinkers, those screening positive for anxiety, and those with less active coping skills. Nicotine dependence was lower among those with medium or low spirituality and among those who exercised moderately or vigorously. Nicotine dependence was almost three times as likely among those who were heavy drinkers compared with those who were not, twice as likely among those who used illicit drugs in the past month as those who did not, and almost twice as likely among risk-takers and smokers compared to those who were not. Nicotine dependence was not related to age, family status, presence of children, combat exposure, region, illness or injury, screening positive for depression or PTSD, and high work or family stress.

Among these measures of substance abuse consequences, which may indicate long-term heavy or problematic use of alcohol or tobacco, significant predictors were substance use and risk-taking. Deployment or combat exposure was not related to any of the measures of substance use consequences, although it had been a significant predictor for the measures of substance use. Illness and injury were related to serious alcohol consequences but not to alcohol dependence or nicotine dependence. Mental health indicators were strong predictors of negative consequences related to substance abuse: serious alcohol consequences were related to screening positive for depression or PTSD, while alcohol dependence was related to screening positive for PTSD, and nicotine dependence was related to screening positive for anxiety.

3.5 Summary and Discussion

Substance use and related consequences have long been problems for the military and can significantly detract from the workplace productivity and physical and mental readiness of military personnel and their ability to meet the challenges placed upon them. With the increased stresses on military personnel that have come with repeated deployments and combat exposure and the need for a highly productive military work force to meet these demands, substance use, and related consequences are now even more critical issues for the military. Because military conditions may exacerbate the problem of substance abuse for the military, substance use remains a significant concern for the armed forces.

3.5.1 Substance Use

In 2008, 12 % of active duty military personnel used illicit drugs, 20 % were heavy drinkers, and 31 % smoked cigarettes in the past month. Rates of illicit drug use overall were lower among military personnel than civilians, although the misuse of prescription drugs was higher among military personnel than civilians. The overall lower rates of illicit drug use among military personnel likely reflect the stringent military policies of zero tolerance for drug abuse that are buttressed by drug testing. Recent increases in illicit drug use among military personnel are largely attributable to increases in misuse of prescription pain relievers, perhaps to ease pain related to high rates of injury among military personnel consistent with findings by Bray et al. (2012). Rates of heavy drinking were higher among military personnel than civilians, while rates of cigarette smoking were similar among the two populations. However, military and civilian differences in substance use vary by age group, with rates of illicit drug use being higher among older military personnel than civilians, rates of heavy drinking being higher among younger military personnel than civilians, and smoking being lower among older military personnel than civilians, in contrast to the general patterns for all ages. These differences may reflect cohort differences or the effects of military policies designed to combat use of these substances.

An IOM committee that examined substance use disorders in the military concluded that "alcohol and other drug use in the armed forces remain unacceptably high, constitute a public health crisis, and both are detrimental to force readiness and psychological fitness" (IOM, 2012). To address these issues, the report asserts that the "highest levels of military leadership must acknowledge these alarming facts and combat them using an arsenal of public health strategies, including proactively attacking substance use problems before they begin by limiting access to certain medications and alcohol" (IOM, 2012). Clearly, the military faces challenges to address these substance use concerns.

Military personnel are predominantly young and male, characteristics generally associated with higher rates of substance use. However, results of logistic regression analyses that controlled for a number of sociodemographic, psychosocial, military, and other characteristics showed that illicit drug use including prescription drug misuse was greater among women than men, while heavy drinking and smoking were greater among men than women. The higher rate of drug use by women is surprising in that men are typically considered at higher risk for drug use. Further examination of drug use rates excluding prescription drugs (Bray, Pemberton et al., 2009) showed that rates for men were similar to or slightly higher than rates for women, suggesting that the higher rates for women noted here are accounted for by misuse of prescription drugs. Illicit drug use was not related to age group, while heavy drinking and smoking were more common among persons aged 21–34 than among other age groups. Among the strongest predictors of all three types of substances were use of other substances, enlisted rank, risk-taking, and deployment and combat exposure. The latter point to the toll taken on personnel from combat deployments and suggest an increased need for substance use services for returning veterans consisted with observations from the recent IOM study of substance use disorders in the military (IOM, 2012).

Among the mental health measures, a significant predictor of illicit drug use and heavy drinking was screening positive for PTSD; significant predictors of heavy drinking and cigarette use included high work or family stress; and a significant predictor of cigarette use was screening positive for depression. Together, these findings point to the comorbid relationship of substance use, stress, and mental health problems. Further, they offer support for the self-medication hypothesis, namely that service members experiencing stress or mental health problems may be turning to substance use as a possible way of coping with these problems.

Experiencing illness and injury were predictors of illicit drug use but not heavy drinking or smoking. A possible explanation for the relationship of illness and injury to illicit drug use may be greater prescription drug misuse and particularly pain medication misuse among military personnel who have extended illnesses or who have been injured.

If prescription drug misuse is excluded, illicit drug misuse is at very low levels, about 2 %. However, prescription drug misuse, binge and heavy drinking, and cigarette smoking remain substantial problems for the military.

Age and pay grade were among the strongest predictors of illicit drug use, heavy alcohol use, and cigarette use, with use concentrated among younger persons and junior pay grades. Also implicated in all three substance use measures were risk-taking and having been deployed or exposed to combat. Screening positive for PTSD was also a significant predictor of illicit drug use and heavy drinking. These findings suggest that substance abuse preventive efforts should be targeted at younger military personnel who also may be greater risk-takers. Substance abuse and PTSD are highly correlated and may occur after deployment; deployed service members are at increased risk of heavy drinking and alcohol-related problems after deployment (Jacobson et al., 2008). Combat exposure has also been implicated in increased risk-taking behavior following deployment, including increased drinking (Killgore et al., 2008).

3.5.2 Consequences of Substance Use

In 2008, 8.7 % of military personnel experienced serious consequences related to alcohol use, 3.8 % experienced alcohol dependence, and 8.3 % experienced nicotine dependence. Serious alcohol consequences decreased during the 1980s and 1990s but have shown a recent increase; alcohol dependence and nicotine dependence showed slight but nonsignificant increases between 2005 and 2008, the two survey years for which data on those two measures were available.

Logistic regression analyses for the substance use consequences measures revealed some predictors in common with the substance use measures but also some differences. Similar to heavy alcohol use, serious consequences of alcohol use were more common among males, younger persons, persons screening positive for PTSD, and risk-takers, but serious consequences of alcohol use were not related to deployment or combat exposure or high work or family stress. Similar to heavy alcohol use, alcohol dependence was more common among men, those screening positive for PTSD, and risk-takers, but was not related to deployment or combat exposure. Similar to smoking, nicotine dependence was more common among males and among risk-takers, but was not related to deployment or combat exposure or to screening positive for PTSD; in contrast to smoking, nicotine dependence was not related to screening positive for depression. Thus, alcohol-related serious consequences and alcohol dependence were related to screening positive for PTSD, but nicotine dependence was not. None of these measures of risky alcohol use or dependence on alcohol or nicotine was related to deployment or combat exposure although the measures of illicit drug use, heavy alcohol use, and cigarette use were related to deployment or combat exposure. The measures of alcohol dependence and nicotine dependence are indicative of longer-term heavy use of these substances.

3.6 Recap

Although there have been long-term declines in illicit drug use and cigarette smoking, heavy alcohol use has been more stable but showed increases from 1998 to 2008, as did binge drinking. Substance abuse remains problematic for military productivity and readiness. Recent increases in illicit drug use appear to be related to misuse of prescription drugs, notably pain relievers, and military personnel are more likely than civilians to misuse prescription drugs. Illicit drug use, heavy alcohol use, and smoking among military personnel are strongly related to use of other substances, enlisted rank, risk-taking propensities and to having been deployed or having combat exposure. Screening positive for PTSD was also predictive of illicit drug use and heavy drinking. Serious consequences related to substance use were also more common among risk-takers, but deployment and combat experience were not related to serious consequences. These findings point to the need for further efforts to prevent substance use and to address the negative effects of risk-taking behaviors, deployment and combat experience, and screening positive for PTSD among military personnel.

References

Ames, G., & Cunradi, C. (2006). *Alcohol use and preventing alcohol-related problems among young adults in the military*. Rockville, MD: NIAAA Publications.

Ames, G. M., Cunradi, C. B., & Moore, R. S. (2002). Alcohol, tobacco, and drug use among young adults prior to entering the military. *Prevention Science, 3*(2), 135–144.

Bachman, J. G., Freedman-Doan, P., O'Malley, P. M., Johnston, L. D., & Segal, D. R. (1999). Changing patterns of drug use among US military recruits before and after enlistment. *American Journal of Public Health, 89*(5), 672–677.

Bray, R. M., Brown, J. M., & Williams, J. (2013). Trends in binge and heavy drinking and alcohol consumption-related problems: Implications of combat exposure in the U.S. Military. *Substance Use and Misuse, 48*(10), 799–810. doi:10.3109/10826084.2013.796990.

Bray, R. M., & Hourani, L. L. (2007). Substance use trends among active duty military personnel: Findings from the united states department of defense health related behavior surveys, 1980–2005. *Addiction, 102*, 1092–1101.

Bray, R. M., Hourani, L. L., Rae Olmsted, K. L., Witt, M., Brown, J. M., Pemberton, M. R., et al. (2006). *2005 Department of Defense survey of health related behaviors among active duty military personnel* (RTI/7841/106-FR). Research Triangle Park, NC: Research Triangle Institute.

Bray, R. M., Marsden, M. E., Herbold, J. R., & Peterson, M. R. (1992). Progress toward eliminating drug and alcohol abuse among military personnel. *Armed Forces and Society, 18*(4), 476–496.

Bray, R. M., Marsden, M. E., Mazzuchi, J. F., & Hartman, R. W. (2009). Prevention in the military. In R. E. Tarter, R. T. Ammerman, & P. J. Ott (Eds.), *Prevention and societal impact of drug and alcohol abuse* (pp. 345–367). Mahwah, NJ: Lawrence Erlbaum Associates.

Bray, R. M., Marsden, M. E., & Peterson, M. R. (1991). Standardized comparisons of the use of alcohol, drugs, and cigarettes among military personnel and civilians. *American Journal of Public Health, 81*, 865–869.

Bray, R. M., Pemberton, M. R., Hourani, L. L., Witt, M., Rae Olmsted, K. L., Brown, J. M., et al. (2009). *2008 Department of Defense survey of health related behaviors among active duty military personnel*. Report prepared for TRICARE Management Activity, Office of the Assistant Secretary of Defense (Health Affairs) and U.S. Coast Guard. Research Triangle Park, NC: Research Triangle Institute.

Bray, R. M., Pemberton, M., Lane, M. E., Hourani, L. L., Mattiko, M., & Babeu, L. A. (2010). Substance use and mental health trends among U.S. Military active duty personnel: Key findings from the 2008 DoD health behavior survey. *Military Medicine, 175*(6), 390–399.

Bray, R. M., Rae Olmsted, K. L., & Williams, J. (2012). Misuse of prescription pain medications in U.S. Active duty service members. In B. K. Wiederhold (Ed.), *Pain syndromes: From recruitment to returning troops* (NATO science for peace and security series E: Human and societal dynamics, Vol. 91, pp. 3–16). Amsterdam, Netherlands: IOS Press.

Centers for Disease Control and Prevention. (2010). Vital signs: Current cigarette smoking among adults aged ≥ 18 years—United States, 2009. *Morbidity and Mortality Weekly, 59*(35), 1135–1140.

Department of Defense. (1970, October 23). *Directive no. 1300.11. Illegal or improper use of drugs by members of the Department of Defense.* Washington, DC: U.S. Department of Defense.

Department of Defense. (1972, March). *Directive no. 1010.2. Alcohol abuse by personnel of the Department of Defense.* Washington, DC: U.S. Department of Defense.

Department of Defense. (1980a). *Directive no. 1010.4. Alcohol and drug abuse by DoD personnel.* Washington, DC: Deputy Secretary of Defense. Reissued September 3, 1997.

Department of Defense. (1980b). *Instruction no. 1010.5. Education and training in alcohol and drug abuse prevention.* Washington, DC: U.S. Department of Defense.

Department of Defense. (1986, March 11). *Directive no. 1010.10. Health promotion.* Washington, DC: U.S. Department of Defense.

Department of Health and Human Services. (2010). *How tobacco smoke causes disease: The biology and behavioral basis for smoking-attributable disease: A report of the surgeon general.* Atlanta, GA: U.S. Department of Health and Human Services, Centers for Disease Control and Prevention, National Center for Chronic Disease and Health Promotion, Office on Smoking and Health.

Department of Health and Human Services. (2012). *About healthy people.* Retrieved from http://www.healthypeople.gov/2020/about/default.aspx

Institute of Medicine (IOM). (2012). *Substance use disorders in the U.S. Armed forces.* Washington, DC: The National Academies Press.

Jacobson, I. G., Ryan, M. A. K., Hooper, T. I., Smith, T. C., Amoroso, P. J., Boyko, E. J., et al. (2008). Alcohol use and alcohol-related problems before and after military combat deployment. *Journal of the American Medical Association, 300*(6), 663–675.

Killgore, W. D. S., Cotting, D. I., Thomas, J. L., Cox, A. L., McGurk, D., Vo, A. H., et al. (2008). Post-combat invincibility: Violent combat experiences are associated with increased risk-taking propensity following deployment. *Journal of Psychiatric Research, 42*(13), 1112–1121.

Mattiko, M., Rae Olmsted, K. L., Brown, J. M., & Bray, R. M. (2011). Alcohol use and negative consequences among active duty military personnel. *Addictive Behaviors, 36*, 608–614.

McGinnis, J. M., Williams-Russo, P., & Knickman, J. R. (2002). The case for more active policy attention to health promotion. *Health Affairs, 21*(2), 78–93.

National Institute on Alcohol Abuse and Alcoholism. (2000). Health risks and benefits of alcohol consumption. *Alcohol Research and Health, 24*(1), 5–11.

National Institute on Drug Abuse. (2011a). *Topics in brief: Substance abuse among the military, veterans, and their families*. Bethesda, MD: National Institute on Drug Abuse.

Schneider Institute for Health Policy. (2001). *Substance abuse: The nation's number one health problem: Key indicators for policy*. Princeton, NJ: Robert Wood Johnson Foundation.

Substance Abuse and Mental Health Services Administration. (2005, November 10). *Substance use, dependence, and treatment among veterans*. The NSDUH Report. www.samhsa.gov/data/2k5/vets/vets.pdf.

Substance Abuse and Mental Health Services Administration. (2011a). *Results from the 2010 national survey on drug use and health: Detailed tables*. Retrieved from http://www.samhsa.www.samhsa.gov/data/NSDUH/2010SummNatFindDetTables/Index.aspx.

Substance Abuse and Mental Health Services Administration. (2011b). *Results from the 2010 national survey on drug use and health: Summary of national findings* (NSDUH Series H-41, HHS Publication No. (SMA) 11-4658). Rockville, MD: Substance Abuse and Mental Health Services Administration.

U.S. Department of Health, Education, and Welfare. (1979). *Healthy people: The surgeon general's report on health promotion and disease prevention*. Washington, DC: U.S. GPO.

U.S. Department of the Army. (2012). *Army 2020: Generating health and discipline in the force ahead of the strategic reset*. Washington, DC: Department of the Army.

Williams, J. O., Bell, N. S., & Amoroso, P. J. (2002). Drinking and other risk behaviors of enlisted male soldiers in the U. S. Army. *Work, 18*(2), 141–150.

Chapter 4
Health Behaviors and Health Status

4.1 Overview and Background

This chapter focuses on healthy lifestyles and health promotion among active duty military personnel with an emphasis on exercise, overweight and obesity status, nutrition, injury, and illness. It examines the behavior of active duty military personnel using selected criteria set by *Healthy People 2010* (Department of Health and Human Services [DHHS], 2000). Data are drawn from the 1995, 1998, 2002, 2005, and 2008 Department of Defense (DoD) Surveys of Health Related Behaviors Among Active Duty Military Personnel (HRB surveys) (Bray, Hourani, et al., 2006; Bray et al., 1995, 1999, 2003, 2009, 2010).

4.1.1 Healthy Lifestyles

Many factors affect the health status of military personnel. Personnel may be exposed to disease and risk of illness and injury in the performance of their duties. Further, personnel's health may be compromised by lifestyle behaviors such as poor nutrition; lack of exercise; becoming overweight; or use of alcohol, tobacco, or illicit drugs. In the United States, heart disease is the leading cause of death, accounting for 25.0 % of total deaths (Heron, 2012) and is impacted by overweight and lack of exercise. The Surgeon General considers tobacco use to be the most important preventable cause of death and disease in the United States (Office on Smoking and Health, 1989). More than one in four deaths in the United States each year can be attributed to the use of alcohol, tobacco, or illicit drugs (Horgan, Skwara, & Strickler, 2001). Many health benefits can be gained by such positive health behaviors as regular physical activity, weight control, and avoiding substance abuse.

The health benefits of exercise and physical fitness are well known. In 1995, the Centers for Disease Control and Prevention (CDC) and the American College of Sports Medicine (ACSM) published physical activity recommendations for public

R.M. Bray et al., *Understanding Military Workforce Productivity: Effects of Substance Abuse, Health, and Mental Health*, DOI 10.1007/978-0-387-78303-1_4,
© Springer Science+Business Media New York 2014

health. The report stated that adults should get at least 30 min of moderate-intensity physical activity on most days, if not every day (DHHS & USDA, 2005). In 1996, *Physical activity and health: A report of the Surgeon General* supported this same recommendation (DHHS, 1996). To track the percentage of adults meeting this guideline, CDC specified that "most" days meant 5 days a week. Since 1995, the common recommendation has been that adults obtain at least 30 min of moderate-intensity physical activity on 5 or more days a week, for a total of at least 150 min a week. In 2008, DHHS issued its first Physical Activity Guidelines for Americans (Subcommittee of the President's Council on Fitness, Sports & Nutrition, 2012) urging regular exercise, which can be a combination of moderate and vigorous levels, to improve health. The Physical Activity Guidelines for Americans affirm that it is acceptable to follow the CDC/ACSM recommendation and similar recommendations. However, the DHHS report indicated that the CDC/ACSM guidelines were too specific and do not allow researchers to say whether the health benefits of 30 min on 5 days a week are any different from the health benefits of 50 min on 3 days a week. As a result, the new guidelines allow a person to accumulate 150 min a week in various ways. Data from the Behavioral Risk Factor Surveillance System indicate that 50 % of men and 47 % of women met the guidelines in 2005, which reflects a slight improvement from the rates in 2001 (48 % of men, 43 % of women). Not surprisingly, physical activity declines with increasing age (CDC, 2007).

In a review of the physical fitness literature among new Army recruits between 1975 and 2003, Knapik et al. (2006) noted that the recruits' physical fitness depended on the component of exercise being measured. For example, muscle *strength* increased from 1978 to 1998, but there was no change in muscle *endurance* between 1984 and 2003. Recruits also exhibited slower times in 1- and 2-mile runs. The authors speculated that this negative trend could be the result of multiple factors, such as increased body weight, inexperience with running, lower motivation, or other environmental factors.

Maintaining healthy body weight has become problematic for both civilian and military populations. Flegal (2005) reported that between 1960 and 1980 the prevalence of overweight and obese adults in the United States was relatively stable but began to increase in the mid-1980s and continued to rise. More recent national estimates (2007–2008) of overweight and obesity indicated that 33.8 % of Americans ages 20 and older were obese (body mass index [BMI] ≥ 30) and 68.0 % were overweight or obese (BMI ≥ 25) (Flegal, Carroll, Ogden, & Curtin, 2010). Although the rate of increase appears to have decelerated (Flegal et al., 2010), the fact that over two in three Americans are overweight or obese is concerning. Increases in weight among military personnel parallel those noted in the general public (Bray, Rae Olmsted, Williams, Sanchez, & Hartzell, 2006; Knapik et al., 2006; Mokdad et al., 1999). For example, Bray, Hourani, et al. (2006) found that the percentage of overweight active duty personnel increased from 49 % in 1995 to 57 % in 2002. These weight increases have serious implications for the efficiency of the military particularly in light of findings that show that excess body weight has been attributed to an estimated 28.4 lost workdays per year for active duty personnel in the Air Force (Robbins, Chao, Russ, & Fonseca, 2002).

Use of alcohol, tobacco, and illicit drugs also has substantial implications for the health of military personnel. Excessive alcohol use, including underage drinking, binge drinking, and heavy drinking, impairs good judgment, is associated with social/family disruptions, and increases the risk of health problems such as injuries, fatal motor-vehicle accidents, physical assault, aggressive behavior, violence, risky sexual behaviors, liver diseases, and cancer (Greenfield, 1998; National Center on Addiction and Substance Abuse at Columbia University, 1999; Smith, Branas, & Miller, 1999; Wechsler, Davenport, Dowdall, Moeykens, & Castillo, 1994). The negative health effects of tobacco use have been well documented and indicate that smoking harms nearly every organ of the body. Specifically, it reduces overall health and causes many diseases, including heart disease, stroke, respiratory disease (bronchitis, emphysema), and various forms of cancer such as lung, bladder, esophageal, kidney, oral, and stomach cancer (DHHS, 2004). Like alcohol and tobacco use, illicit drug use is associated with many harmful behaviors and can cause both short- and long-term health problems. Young people who use illicit drugs are more likely to engage in risky sexual behavior (Kaiser Foundation, 2002), to have poor relationships with their families and peers (Office of National Drug Control Policy [ONDCP], 2003), to engage in delinquency and crime (Wilson, 2000; Windle & Mason, 2004), and to drop out of school or be expelled (McCluskey, Krohn, Lizotte, & Rodriguez, 2002; National Center on Addiction and Substance Abuse at Columbia University, 2001). Illicit drug use is associated with numerous health problems, which vary depending on the type of drug used. Physical problems can include abnormal heart rates, seizures, kidney failure, respiratory failure, and brain damage (ONDCP, 2003). A variety of mental health problems are also linked to illicit drug use, including depression, anxiety, paranoia, hallucinations, developmental lags, delusions, and mood disturbances (Crowe & Bilchik, 1998).

Illness and injuries are also of considerable concern to military leadership because they negatively impact the readiness and productivity of the armed forces. Illnesses from a medical perspective can be defined as the presence of symptoms that can range from mild to severe, whereas health can be defined as the absence of symptoms. The leading reasons for outpatient visits in civilian settings are symptoms of back pain, headache, gastrointestinal disturbance, musculoskeletal pain, fatigue, dizziness, and other physical complaints (Green & Pope, 1999; Kroenke & Spitzer, 1998). Patients also have symptoms associated with well-defined diseases. All illnesses reduce the functionality and capability of service members to engage in their peacetime and wartime duties, but this is especially true for serious illnesses. Illness and military service are two sides of the same coin. Illness reduces readiness for military duty, but military service can increase the risk for subsequent disease as has occurred with some environmental exposures during combat. For example, studies of exposure to Agent Orange, a blend of herbicides used during the Vietnam War, show a positive association to a variety of subsequent diseases. These include soft-tissue sarcoma (including heart), lymphoma, and several forms of leukemia. Other studies show a less definitive but suggestive association of herbicide exposure and cancers of the larynx, lung, bronchus, trachea, and prostate, and certain birth defects of veterans' biological children (Institute of Medicine [IOM],

2010a). Similarly, following service in the Gulf War in 1991, many veterans reported unexplained symptoms that collectively have been called Gulf War Syndrome. About one-fourth of the 700,000 veterans who served in the 1991 Gulf War developed symptoms that include chronic headaches, widespread pain, memory and concentration problems, persistent fatigue, gastrointestinal problems, skin abnormalities, and mood disturbances. Although exposed military personnel have exhibited a cluster of symptoms, the studies of Gulf War Syndrome have shown conflicting results regarding whether these were a result of chemical exposure. An IOM committee concluded that current evidence is inadequate to determine whether an association exists between multi-symptom illness and any specific battlefield exposure or exposures (IOM, 2010b).

Injuries have been identified as the single most significant medical impediment to military readiness (Jones, Amoroso, Canham, Weyandt, & Schmitt, 1999) and the largest health problem faced by the military (Jones, Canham-Chervak, & Sleet, 2010). Injuries are very costly and represent a complex problem that impacts the military's strength and ability to respond to its mission. Despite the importance of injuries, only very recently have the nature and extent of the injury problem been recognized. In 1994, the Armed Forces Epidemiological Board formed the Injury Prevention and Control Work Group and charged it with (a) examining the size and extent of injuries in the military services, (b) determining the information systems that exist to support a comprehensive integrated injury prevention and control effort, and (c) identifying what needs to be done to more effectively prevent injuries in the military. The work group produced a report that identified injuries as "a hidden epidemic" in the military and concluded that "injuries have a greater impact on the health and readiness of U.S. armed forces than any other category of medical complaint during peacetime and combat" (Jones & Hansen, 1996). The work group developed recommendations about improvements in injury surveillance, research on injuries, and prevention of injuries. They further prepared a comprehensive atlas of injuries in the military and urged that a public health approach be followed to prevent and reduce military injuries (Jones et al., 1999; Jones, Perrotta, Canham-Chervak, Nee, & Brundage, 2000).

In 2007, DoD reported that there were 2.1 million injury-related medical visits affecting 900,000 service members. Further, injuries were ranked as the second most common cause of hospitalizations, accounting for almost 110,000 days in the hospital and were classified as the leading cause of outpatient clinical visits. Musculoskeletal injuries were responsible for 68 % of all limited-duty days and medical profiles, which resulted in an estimated 25 million limited-duty days per year (McNulty, 2009).

Injuries range from minor to life-threatening with the most serious resulting in death. Table 4.1 presents data on reasons for deaths from 1980 to 2010 among active duty personnel. As shown, accidents (often from motor vehicle crashes) were the leading cause of death, accounting for half of or more of all military deaths from 1980 to 2000. Accidents continued to be a leading cause of death and were exceeded only by death by hostile actions from 2004 to 2010.

Table 4.1 Percentages and numbers of military deaths by category, 1980–2010

	Year											
	1980	1990	1995	2000	2004	2005	2006	2007	2008	2009	2010	Total
Category (percentage)												
Accidents	65.1	58.4	51.7	51.1	32.4	33.4	29.8	28.7	34.8	30.5	27.4	40.0
Hostile action	0.0	0.0	0.0	0.0	39.4	38.0	40.8	43.4	24.4	22.8	30.7	23.8
Homicides	7.3	4.9	6.4	4.4	2.5	2.8	2.5	2.7	3.3	5.1	2.4	4.0
Illnesses	17.5	18.4	16.7	21.5	14.5	15.0	13.7	12.1	16.8	18.0	15.8	16.0
Suicides	9.7	15.4	24.0	18.9	10.8	9.4	11.3	10.8	17.9	19.0	18.3	14.0
Other[a]	0.5	2.9	1.1	4.0	0.5	1.4	1.9	2.4	2.8	4.6	5.4	2.3
Total	100.0	100.0	100.0	100.0	100.0	100.0	100.0	100.0	100.0	100.0	100.0	100.0
Category (numbers)												
Accidents	1,556	880	538	430	607	648	561	560	501	462	406	7,149
Hostile action	0	0	0	0	738	739	768	847	351	346	455	4,244
Homicides	174	74	67	37	46	54	47	52	47	77	36	711
Illnesses	419	277	174	181	272	291	257	237	242	273	235	2,858
Suicides	231	232	250	159	202	183	213	211	257	288	271	2,497
Other[a]	12	44	11	34	9	28	35	46	41	69	80	409
Total	2,392	1,507	1,040	841	1,874	1,943	1,881	1,953	1,439	1,515	1,483	17,868

Source: Department of Defense Personnel and Procurement, DoD Personnel and Military Casualty Statistics, "Military Information," http://siadapp.dmdc.osd.mil/personnel/CASUALTY/castop.htm
Note: Top portion of table displays the percentages of deaths by category per year. Bottom portion of table displays the associated numbers of deaths per category per year.
[a]Includes all deaths that are pending, undetermined, or related to terrorist attacks

4.1.2   DoD Health Directives

DoD has had a long-standing interest in the health and well-being of its members because of the positive effects of sound health practices and the importance of good health for military productivity and readiness. Indeed, having ready access to a comprehensive health care program at little or no cost to service members has long been viewed as an important benefit of military life (Stanley & Blair, 1993). Health promotion efforts in the military emerged as an outgrowth of drug and alcohol abuse problems that surfaced in the 1970s. In response to reports of widespread drug abuse among troops during the Vietnam War, and in recognition of the significance of the alcohol abuse problem in the services, DoD issued a policy directive in March 1972 (Directive No. 1010.2, DoD, 1972) that set forth prevention and treatment policies for alcohol abuse and alcoholism among military personnel. Other DoD policy directives (e.g., DoD Directive Nos. 1010.3 and 1010.4 and Instruction Nos. 1010.5 and 1010.6, DoD, 1980a, 1980b, 1985a, 1985b) and programs further amplified and expanded these efforts. These additional directives provide for (a) assessment of the nature, extent, and consequences of substance use and abuse in the military (DoD, 1980a, 1985b, 1997); (b) prevention programs designed to deter substance abuse, which include both education and drug urinalysis testing (DoD, 1980b); (c) treatment and rehabilitation programs designed to return substance abusers to full performance capabilities (DoD, 1985a); and (d) evaluation of drug urinalysis programs and treatment and rehabilitation programs (DoD, 1985b, 1997).

In 1986, DoD established a formal, coordinated, and integrated health promotion policy (DoD Directive No. 1010.10) designed to improve and maintain military readiness and the quality of life of DoD personnel and other beneficiaries (DoD, 1986). This directive defined health promotion as activities designed to support and influence individuals to manage their own health through lifestyle decisions and self-care. It identified six broad program areas: smoking prevention and cessation, physical fitness, nutrition, stress management, alcohol and other drug abuse prevention, and hypertension prevention. This directive was updated and reissued in 2003 (DoD, 2003). In response to these directives, each branch of the military established its own health promotion programs to meet the distinctive problems and needs of its members and to focus on improving and maintaining the health of military personnel.

Building on and moving beyond these directives, DoD continues to consider ways to improve the health and fitness of the force. For example, Total Force Fitness is a recent new approach that is being considered that invites a paradigm shift in conceptualizing optimal health. This approach broadens the concept of fitness to include more than the traditional physical domain. In this approach, total fitness encompasses and integrates eight wide-ranging domains: social, behavioral, psychological, nutritional, spiritual, medical, environmental, and physical (Jonas, Deuster, O'Conner, & Macedonia, 2010). Together, these domains make up a comprehensive holistic approach to health. Individual elements of the domains are covered by various programs in one or more of the services, but the challenge is to garner acceptance from critical leaders about the importance of all of these domains, to develop strong metrics for measuring progress, and to change training approaches such that they include and integrate all of the domains. A related thrust for improving the health of the force builds on concepts of worksite health promotion in response to a DoD initiative to improve employee wellness. An analysis by the Defense Centers of Excellence for Psychological Health and Traumatic Brain Injury identified key principles for how to increase the effectiveness of health promotion efforts. This analysis concluded that workforce health promotion programs must consider multiple determinants of health, particularly the relationship between environmental factors and associated health risks (Pinder, Gilbert, Rhodes, Brown, & Bates, 2011).

4.1.3   Healthy People Objectives

Beginning with *Healthy People: The Surgeon General's report on health promotion and disease prevention* (Public Health Service, 1979) and continuing in 1980 with *Promoting health/preventing disease: Objectives for the nation* (Public Health

Service, 1980), the federal government adopted a national health agenda. Broadly speaking, the agenda is aimed at taking steps to prevent unnecessary disease and disability and to achieve a better quality of life for all Americans. These initial efforts were followed by *Healthy People 2000: National health promotion and disease prevention objectives* (Public Health Service, 1991), *Healthy People 2010: Understanding and improving health* (DHHS, 2000), and most recently *Healthy People 2020* (www.healthypeople.gov). The purpose of *Healthy People 2000* was to commit the nation to the attainment of three broad goals during the 1990s: (a) increase the span of healthy life for Americans, (b) reduce health disparities among Americans, and (c) achieve access to preventive services for all Americans. Accordingly, measurable goals or targets were set forth across 28 areas, broadly grouped into four categories: health promotion, health protection, preventive services, and surveillance and data systems. The goal of *Healthy People 2010* was to continue to improve the health of individuals, communities, and the nation by increasing the quality and years of healthy life for all Americans and by eliminating health disparities among segments of the population. *Healthy People 2020* builds on the accomplishments of prior *Healthy People* efforts and is committed to the vision of a society in which all people live long, healthy lives. New features emphasizing health equity address social determinants of health and promote health across all stages of life.

Beginning with the *Healthy People 2000* objectives, DoD identified those most relevant to the military. Of the 383 objectives, 181 were identified as being of initial primary concern to DoD. Of these 181 objectives, 45 were prioritized and designated as being of the highest importance for near-term measurement (Office of the Assistant Secretary of Defense [Health Affairs], 1992). From these 45 objectives, DoD identified a subset that focused on health-related behaviors thought to be measurable with surveys and began to monitor progress toward these objectives with the 1995 and 1998 DoD surveys. The 2002 DoD survey assessed how well the *Healthy People 2000* objectives were met and also served as a baseline measure for *Healthy People 2010* objectives, which continued to be measured with the 2005 and 2008 HRB surveys.

Several studies have examined various military services' achievement of the *Healthy People 2000* objectives of physical fitness and good nutrition. Yore, Bell, Senier, and Amoroso (2000) compared responses from the 1998 U.S. Army Health Risk Appraisal survey to *Healthy People 2000* objectives. These researchers reported that in 1998 U.S. Army personnel exceeded *Healthy People 2000* objectives for physical fitness and eating high-fiber foods but failed to meet some of the nutritional goals. For example, the proportion of Army personnel eating high-fiber foods (52 %) surpassed the *Healthy People 2000* goal of 50 %, while the goals for reducing intake of salt and high-fat foods were not met. When Warber, Boquist, and Cline (1997) estimated the number of servings of fruits and vegetables consumed by active duty service members, they found that military personnel eating in institutional dining facilities met the minimum requirement for fruits (two servings per day) and vegetables (three servings per day) at a higher rate than the general public. On any given day, 57 % of military personnel met the requirement for vegetable consumption, 71 % met the requirement for fruit consumption, and 43 % met both.

Williamson et al. (2002) evaluated changes in food selections, food intake, and body weight during 8 weeks of basic combat training (BCT) and found a trend toward improvement in healthy eating and healthy weight. With the exception of fruits and vegetables, the consumption of most food groups during BCT improved. However, sugar intake was very high in week 1 and increased further by week 8. Despite the increased sugar intake, overweight soldiers lost weight, and thin soldiers gained weight. When Trent and Hurtado (1998) examined eating habits among military personnel, they found highly significant improvement in dietary choices between 1983 and 1989; they also found that women surpassed men in their choices of healthy foods.

In their study of progress toward *Healthy People 2000* objectives for active duty service personnel, Bray, Rae Olmsted, et al. (2006) compared weight, physical activity, and other health indicators from 1995 to 2002. They found that military personnel met or exceeded 7 of 15 selected healthy behaviors and that objectives were most likely to be met in instances where personnel's behaviors were closely monitored. For example, military personnel exceeded the objective for engaging in vigorous exercise, which is not surprising because service members must pass annual physical fitness tests and many units either perform fitness training together or allow personnel time to train during duty hours.

4.1.4   *Achievement of Selected* Healthy People 2010 *Objectives in 2008*

In this section, we report data from the 2008 HRB survey assessing *Healthy People* objectives among active duty service members. Table 4.2 provides the *Healthy People 2010* objectives and the associated prevalence for DoD personnel toward the objectives of tobacco use, binge drinking, illicit drug use, weight levels, exercise, and food intake. As shown, military personnel in 2008 failed to meet *Healthy People* objectives for cigarette smoking, smokeless tobacco use, binge drinking, and illicit drug use. For example, the 2010 objective for cigarette smoking in the past 30 days was 12.0 %, but the military rate in 2008 was considerably above that rate at 30.6 %. Similarly, 47.1 % of military personnel reported binge drinking in the past 30 days compared to a 2010 objective of 6.0 %.

Service members had a higher rate of vigorous exercise than recommended by the *Healthy People 2010* objective. Over 60 % of military personnel in 2008 engaged in vigorous exercise, compared with a *Healthy People 2010* objective of 30 % or more of the nation. In 2010, the objectives for overweight in *Healthy People 2000* were replaced with objectives for healthy weight and obesity although overweight remains a concern. Nearly 62 % of service members were overweight based on BMI criteria whereas only about 40 % were at a healthy weight. It is encouraging, however, that in 2008, military personnel met the *Healthy People 2010* objective of fewer than 15 % of individuals being obese.

Table 4.2 Selected *Healthy People 2010* objectives and prevalence of DoD personnel engaging in behaviors, 2008

Characteristic/group	HP 2010 objective	2008 HRB survey[a]
Any cigarette use, past 30 days	≤12.0	30.6 (1.2)
Smokeless tobacco use, past 30 days	≤0.4	13.6 (0.6)
Binge drinking, past 30 days	≤6.0	47.1 (1.2)
Any Illicit drug use including prescription drug misuse, past 30 days	≤2.0	12.0 (0.4)
Overweight—aged 20 or older	NA[b]	61.8 (0.6)
Obese—aged 20 or older	≤15	13.2 (0.3)
Healthy weight—aged 20 or older	≥60	37.2 (0.6)
Vigorous physical activity, past 30 days	≥30	62.6 (0.9)
Food intake—fruits and vegetables		
Fruits ≥3 times/day	≥75	12.7 (0.5)
Vegetables ≥3 times/day	≥50	14.2 (0.4)

Source: DoD Survey of Health Related Behaviors Among Active Duty Military Personnel, 2008
Note: HRB survey data are the percentages of military personnel who reported the listed characteristic or behavior. The standard error of each estimate is presented in parentheses.
[a]Percentages have not been adjusted for any demographic or other characteristics
[b]*Healthy People 2010* does not have a specific objective for overweight; it was replaced by the objective for healthy weight

The *Healthy People* objective regarding fruit and vegetable consumption was not met. Fewer than 15 % of military personnel consumed fruits and vegetables at adequate levels, compared with objectives of 75 and 50 %, respectively. In addition to the *Healthy People 2010* focus on increased consumption of daily servings of fruits and vegetables, *Healthy People 2010* also recommends a healthful assortment of nutrient dense food types, including whole grains, low-fat dairy products, and lean proteins. The 2005 HRB survey measured the percentages of personnel who consumed these foods as well as other types of grain, dairy, and protein products, snack foods/sweets, and fast foods (Bray, Rae Olmsted, et al., 2006). In the whole grain category, 11.3 % of personnel consumed three or more servings per day, which is far below the *Healthy People 2010* recommendation of 50 %. Low-fat dairy products consumption also was below the *Healthy People 2010* objective of 50 %: only 11.5 % of military personnel reported eating three or more servings per day. Lean protein consumption also was low: 9.4 % of personnel reported eating three or more servings per day. On the plus side, the consumption of three or more servings per day of fast foods also was low (5.3 %) as was consumption of snack foods and sweets (9.7 %). Reported percentages of the consumption of other non-recommended foods, such as unhealthy types of grains and proteins and high-fat dairy products, were consistently lower than the percentages reported for healthful foods (11.3, 7.4, and 7.8 % for unhealthy types of grains, proteins, and dairy products, respectively).

4.2 Trends in Overweight, Illness, and Injury

Figure 4.1 presents findings on trends in overweight, illness, and injury from 1995 to 2008 based on data from the HRB surveys. As shown, overweight (BMI ≥ 25.0) showed a steady increase among active duty DoD personnel from 50 % in 1995 to 60 % in 2005. The rate of overweight remained at the 2005 level in 2008.

To investigate changes in weight further, we examined the trends in overweight (BMI 25.0–29.9) and obesity (BMI 30 or higher) for two age groups, personnel aged less than 20 years and personnel aged 20 or older. These trends are shown in Fig. 4.2 from 1995 through 2008. As shown, across the DoD services for personnel under age 20, the percentage of service members classified as overweight or obese increased from 28 % in 1995 to 45 % in 2005, and then declined to 35 % in 2008. This overall pattern was driven by changes in both the overweight and obese groups. The percentage of personnel classified as obese among persons under 20 was very low in 1995 and 1998 (approximately 1–2 %), increased slightly to 3 % in 2002, rose to 7 % in 2005, and then dropped back to the 1995 level of 3 % in 2008.

For personnel aged 20 or older, the percentage classified as overweight or obese according to BMI increased from 51 % in 1995 to 62 % in 2005, and remained at that same level in 2008. Of interest, most of the overall increase occurred among persons meeting the criteria for obesity. For this age group, the percentage of service members classified as obese rose from 5 % in 1995 to 13 % in 2005 and remained at that level in 2008, whereas those classified as overweight were relatively stable across the period.

One of the explanations for increases in overweight among civilians is that the U.S. population has become more sedentary and fails to exercise at high enough levels.

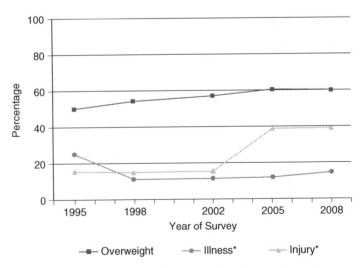

Fig. 4.1 Trends in overweight, illness, and injury among DoD personnel, 1995–2008
*Past 12 months

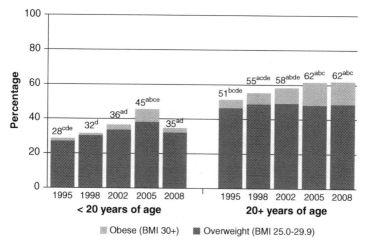

Fig. 4.2 Trends in overweight and obesity among DoD personnel, 1995–2008
[a]Estimate is statistically significant from the 1995 estimate at the 0.05 level
[b]Estimate is statistically significant from the 1998 estimate at the 0.05 level
[c]Estimate is statistically significant from the 2002 estimate at the 0.05 level
[d]Estimate is statistically significant from the 2005 estimate at the 0.05 level
[e]Estimate is statistically significant from the 2008 estimate at the 0.05 level

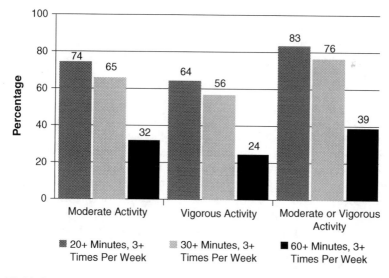

Fig. 4.3 Moderate or vigorous physical activity in the past month among DoD personnel, 2008

This seems less likely in the military, however, because of the military's emphasis
on physical fitness and exercise. Figure 4.3 provides information about the rates of
moderate and vigorous physical activity at least three times per week among active
duty military personnel for three periods of exercise: 20 or more minutes in duration,

Table 4.3 Comparison of exercise and overweight by gender and age group, 2008

Gender/age group	Moderate exercise	Vigorous exercise	Moderate or vigorous exercise	Overweight (BMI 25+)
Males				
20 or younger	76.2 (1.2)	70.8 (1.9)	84.3 (1.4)	40.6 (1.2)
21–24	76.2 (1.2)	66.1* (1.2)	83.1 (1.1)	54.1* (1.0)
25–34	77.7 (0.6)	66.8* (1.0)	85.5 (0.6)	69.4* (0.8)
35–44	72.3* (1.0)	61.5* (1.1)	82.2 (0.8)	78.0* (1.0)
45+	70.1* (1.9)	59.0* (1.6)	81.2 (1.6)	77.2* (2.1)
Total male	75.7 (0.6)	65.8 (0.9)	83.8 (0.6)	63.5 (0.7)
Females				
20 or younger	75.3 (2.5)	57.4 (2.8)	81.9 (1.8)	27.7 (2.5)
21–24	72.0 (1.2)	56.2 (2.2)	80.5 (1.4)	35.3* (2.2)
25–34	74.9 (1.3)	56.1 (1.9)	82.5 (1.5)	43.5* (1.6)
35–44	73.3 (1.4)	52.8 (1.5)	81.8 (1.5)	53.5* (2.2)
45+	69.6 (3.6)	52.6 (6.3)	75.2 (3.1)	48.6* (3.4)
Total female	73.6 (0.9)	55.7 (1.3)	81.4 (1.0)	40.2 (1.2)
Total across genders by age				
20 or younger	76.0 (1.2)	68.6 (1.9)	83.9 (1.3)	38.5 (1.2)
21–24	75.5 (1.1)	64.5* (1.3)	82.7 (1.00)	50.9* (0.9)
25–34	77.3 (0.5)	65.3 (1.0)	85.1 (0.5)	65.8* (0.8)
35–44	72.4* (0.9)	60.5* (1.1)	82.1 (0.8)	75.1* (1.1)
45+	70.1* (1.6)	58.1* (1.7)	80.3 (1.3)	73.2* (2.0)
Total across ages	75.4 (0.6)	64.3 (0.9)	83.5 (0.6)	60.1 (0.7)

Source: DoD Survey of Health Related Behaviors Among Active Duty Military Personnel, 2008
Note: Table shows percentages with standard errors of military personnel by gender and age who reported moderate and vigorous physical activity 3 or more days a week for at least 20 min per occasion.
*Estimate is significantly different from the personnel aged 20 or younger

30 or more minutes in duration, and 60 or more minutes in duration. As might be expected, higher percentages of personnel engaged in moderate activity than in vigorous activity and service members were more likely to exercise for shorter periods of time than for longer periods. In 2008, an estimated 83 % of personnel indicated that they got 20 min or more of moderate or vigorous physical activity at least 3 times per week. Three out of four personnel (76 %) indicated getting 30 min or more, and 39 % reported getting 60 min or more of moderate or vigorous physical activity at least three times per week. Although personnel were less likely to engage in more intense exercise, still about two thirds of personnel reported vigorous activity for at least 20 min or more three times per week.

Table 4.3 further examines this issue for the military by comparing how exercise and overweight vary for military men and women by age group. As shown, 65.8 % of men reported engaging in vigorous exercise during the past month, and 83.8 % reported moderate or vigorous exercise. The 55.7 % rate of vigorous exercise among military women was lower than for men, but the 81.4 % rate of moderate or vigorous exercise was similar to that for men. There was a pattern of less vigorous exercise as age increased (68.6–58.1 %), but less change for a combination of moderate or vigorous exercise over the age span. There was no statistical difference in the likelihood of moderate or vigorous exercise between those who were aged 45 or older (80.3 %) and those who were 20 or younger (83.9 %).

Despite relatively high rates of moderate or vigorous exercise among military service members, overweight showed a clear linear increase with age. Those who were older were more likely to be overweight than those who were younger. Of interest, the rates of overweight for the top two age groups (35–44 and 45+) were about the same for men, which suggests that overweight peaked in the 35–44 age range. Women also showed the highest rate of overweight in the 35–44 age group and showed a decrease among those 45 and older. Men were substantially more likely to be overweight (65.2 %) than women (41.3 %).

Returning to the trends in illness and injury shown in Fig. 4.1, the rate of illness declined from about 25.1 % in 1995 to 11.1 % in 1998, remained at that level in 2002 and 2005, and then increased to 14.6 % in 2008. In contrast, injury rates were relatively low in 1995 at 15.4 %, and remained at that level in 1998 and 2002, but then showed a large and notable increase to 38.8 % in 2005 and remained at this higher level in 2008.

4.3 Correlates and Predictors of Healthy Behaviors for 2008

To identify those military populations at greatest risk for overweight or obesity, illness, and injury, and to examine potential protective factors for these outcomes, a series of logistic models were conducted that estimated odds ratios while controlling for all other variables in the model. These comprehensive models accounted for 10, 12, and 15 % of the total variance in these three outcomes, respectively.

4.3.1 Overweight and Obesity

As shown in Table 4.4, military women (42.7 %) were much less likely to be overweight or obese than military men (66.2 %) as determined by having a BMI of 25 or higher. Age was the strongest predictor of overweight with younger personnel being at much lower risk of being overweight or obese than older personnel. There was a strong increase in the proportion of overweight or obese personnel with each advancing age group (ranging from 43.2 to 73.8 %). Hispanics and African Americans were significantly more likely to be overweight or obese than whites or other racial/ethnic groups. Of interest, unmarried personnel were significantly less likely to be overweight or obese than those who were married and accompanied by their spouse even after controlling for other variables in the model.

In terms of military variables, senior officers were the least likely of all pay grade groups to be overweight or obese after adjusting for other variables in the model

Table 4.4 Correlates of overweight/obese, illness, and injury in past 12 months, 2008

	Overweight/obese (BMI ≥25)			Illness			Injury		
Independent variables	Unadjusted %	Adjusted %	Adjusted ORs[a] (95 % CI)[b]	Unadjusted %	Adjusted %	Adjusted ORs[a] (95 % CI)[b]	Unadjusted %	Adjusted %	Adjusted ORs[a] (95 % CI)[b]
Gender									
Male	65.2	66.2	1.00	13.5	8.1	1.00	49.0	51.3	1.00
Female	41.3	42.7	0.38* (0.34–0.43)	19.1	12.7	1.65* (1.47–1.85)	52.4	54.8	1.15* (1.03–1.29)
Age									
20 or younger	41.2	43.2	0.27* (0.21–0.34)	12.6	7.9	0.82 (0.58–1.17)	40.3	41.7	0.45* (0.36–0.55)
21–25	52.1	53.7	0.41* (0.35–0.48)	15.1	8.6	0.90 (0.71–1.15)	48.1	46.4	0.54* (0.47–0.62)
26–34	67.0	66.6	0.71* (0.60–0.83)	14.0	8.2	0.86 (0.73–1.02)	49.9	51.5	0.66* (0.59–0.74)
35 or older	74.8	73.8	1.00	14.7	9.4	1.00	56.5	61.6	1.00
Race/ethnicity									
White non-Hispanic	59.9	60.9	0.75* (0.67–0.84)	13.2	8.2	0.82* (0.68–0.98)	50.0	53.2	1.14 (0.98–1.32)
African American non-Hispanic	67.4	67.6	1.00	16.7	9.8	1.00	50.4	49.9	1.00
Hispanic	67.8	71.5	1.20* (1.04–1.40)	15.8	9.1	0.92 (0.77–1.12)	46.4	47.3	0.90 (0.72–1.13)
Other	57.8	59.3	0.70* (0.62–0.80)	16.1	9.9	1.01 (0.79–1.31)	48.0	49.9	1.00 (0.85–1.17)
Family status									
Not married	54.1	60.5	0.82* (0.73–0.91)	13.8	8.5	1.01 (0.84–1.21)	46.5	50.6	0.91 (0.79–1.04)
Married–spouse not present	62.8	60.9	0.83 (0.68–1.02)	17.7	10.3	1.24 (1.00–1.53)	51.8	50.0	0.88 (0.74–1.05)
Married–spouse present	68.1	65.1	1.00	14.1	8.5	1.00	51.9	53.1	1.00
Children living with you									
Yes	69.3	64.0	1.08 (0.98–1.19)	15.5	9.3	1.14 (0.96–1.36)	53.1	50.7	0.92 (0.82–1.04)
No	56.4	62.1	1.00	13.5	8.2	1.00	47.2	52.7	1.00
Pay grade									
E1–E3	49.4	65.5	1.94* (1.63–2.31)	14.6	9.9	1.85* (1.29–2.67)	44.0	51.7	1.08 (0.85–1.38)
E4–E6	61.6	63.2	1.76* (1.51–2.05)	15.8	9.5	1.78* (1.26–2.52)	51.6	53.4	1.16 (0.95–1.40)
E7–E9	81.1	70.4	2.43* (1.87–3.16)	14.7	8.0	1.47* (1.10–1.97)	56.1	51.6	1.07 (0.90–1.28)

W1–W5	75.5	65.9	1.97* (1.31–2.99)	16.8	12.3	2.38* (1.54–3.70)	52.1	41.5	0.72* (0.56–0.92)
O1–O3	57.4	57.7	1.39* (1.15–1.69)	8.6	6.2	1.13 (0.80–1.58)	41.5	47.8	0.93 (0.75–1.14)
O4–O10	62.9	49.4	1.00	8.9	5.6	1.00	50.6	49.8	1.00
Service									
Army	63.0	62.0	0.96 (0.86–1.09)	16.7	8.5	1.00 (0.77–1.29)	58.0	59.4	1.67* (1.36–2.05)
Navy	63.6	65.8	1.14* (1.02–1.27)	12.5	8.4	0.98 (0.77–1.24)	41.3	43.7	0.89 (0.74–1.07)
Marine Corps	58.1	59.8	0.88* (0.81–0.96)	16.5	9.6	1.13 (0.94–1.37)	51.9	55.4	1.42* (1.26–1.61)
Air Force	59.9	62.9	1.00	11.1	8.6	1.00	42.6	46.6	1.00
Deployment and combat exposure									
Not deployed	50.9	60.0	0.87* (0.79–0.97)	13.6	9.1	1.31* (1.04–1.65)	45.6	52.8	1.17* (1.01–1.35)
Deployed-none	63.6	63.2	1.00	9.7	7.1	1.00	41.9	48.9	1.00
Deployed-moderate	65.8	63.5	1.01 (0.89–1.14)	12.4	8.0	1.14 (0.93–1.40)	52.1	54.0	1.23* (1.11–1.36)
Deployed-high	68.3	65.1	1.08 (0.92–1.28)	19.3	10.8	1.59* (1.21–2.09)	59.2	51.6	1.11 (0.95–1.30)
Average hours of nightly sleep									
7+ h	57.3	60.1	1.00	10.7	8.1	1.00	42.0	48.9	1.00
5–6 h	62.9	63.3	1.15* (1.03–1.28)	13.3	8.6	1.06 (0.89–1.27)	49.7	51.9	1.13* (1.01–1.25)
4 h or less	64.0	65.9	1.28* (1.08–1.52)	21.5	9.6	1.19 (0.96–1.47)	60.6	56.5	1.35* (1.17–1.57)
Region									
CONUS	61.8	63.0	1.00	15.1	9.1	1.00	50.0	52.3	1.00
OCONUS/Afloats	61.6	62.7	0.99 (0.89–1.10)	12.9	7.8	0.85 (0.71–1.03)	48.5	51.0	0.95 (0.80–1.13)
History of physical/sexual abuse									
Yes	61.4	63.0	1.01 (0.93–1.09)	16.2	8.4	0.96 (0.82–1.11)	56.5	56.5	1.39* (1.28–1.50)
No	61.9	62.8	1.00	12.5	8.8	1.00	44.4	48.4	1.00
Risk-taking/impulsivity									
Yes	56.2	58.7	0.83* (0.69–0.99)	20.4	9.5	1.12 (0.93–1.35)	56.1	55.2	1.16 (0.98–1.37)
No	62.3	63.2	1.00	13.7	8.6	1.00	48.8	51.6	1.00
Spirituality									
High	61.8	61.2	1.00	14.7	9.5	1.00	49.0	50.2	1.00

(continued)

Table 4.4 (continued)

Independent variables	Overweight/obese (BMI ≥25)			Illness			Injury		
	Unadjusted %	Adjusted %	Adjusted ORs[a] (95 % CI)[b]	Unadjusted %	Adjusted %	Adjusted ORs[a] (95 % CI)[b]	Unadjusted %	Adjusted %	Adjusted ORs[a] (95 % CI)[b]
Medium	62.6	63.8	1.12* (1.01–1.24)	13.9	8.3	0.86* (0.75–0.99)	50.1	52.8	1.11* (1.02–1.20)
Low	60.3	62.8	1.07 (0.99–1.16)	13.4	8.4	0.87 (0.72–1.06)	48.8	51.6	1.06 (0.93–1.20)
Moderate/vigorous physical exercise in past month									
Yes	61.9	63.0	1.03 (0.92–1.15)	13.2	8.0	0.61* (0.51–0.73)	49.4	52.0	1.03 (0.94–1.14)
No	61.1	62.3	1.00	19.2	12.5	1.00	50.2	51.2	1.00
Overweight/obese (BMI ≥25)									
Yes	–	–	–	14.8	8.9	1.10 (0.94–1.29)	53.1	54.1	1.27* (1.15–1.39)
No	–	–	–	12.8	8.2	1.00	45.8	48.2	1.00
Illness in past 12 months									
Yes	65.2	64.8	1.10 (0.94–1.29)	–	–	–	87.1	86.1	7.54* (6.30–9.02)
No	61.2	62.6	1.00	–	–	–	43.1	45.1	1.00
Injury in past 12 months									
Yes	65.2	65.6	1.27* (1.15–1.39)	25.2	20.5	7.54* (6.31–9.01)	–	–	–
No	58.3	60.1	1.00	3.7	3.3	1.00	–	–	–
Fruits 3+ times/day									
Yes	59.6	60.6	0.89 (0.80–1.00)	16.6	9.3	1.09 (0.91–1.32)	48.7	51.1	0.97 (0.83–1.12)
No	62.0	63.2	1.00	13.6	8.6	1.00	49.6	52.0	1.00
Vegetables 3+ times/day									
Yes	62.3	65.2	1.12 (0.98–1.27)	16.3	9.0	1.05 (0.87–1.27)	50.4	52.1	1.01 (0.89–1.15)
No	61.6	62.6	1.00	13.6	8.6	1.00	49.4	51.8	1.00
Illicit drug use in past month									
Yes	63.7	63.5	1.03 (0.92–1.14)	24.0	11.7	1.45* (1.20–1.76)	63.1	59.1	1.39* (1.20–1.61)
No	61.5	62.8	1.00	12.9	8.3	1.00	47.7	51.0	1.00

Heavy alcohol use in past month									
Yes	62.6	65.8	1.17* (1.03–1.32)	16.2	8.9	1.04 (0.83–1.29)	53.1	52.6	1.04 (0.94–1.14)
No	61.3	62.2	1.00	13.3	8.6	1.00	48.6	51.7	1.00
Cigarette use in past month									
Yes	58.3	59.1	0.80* (0.74–0.86)	16.2	9.0	1.07 (0.90–1.27)	53.9	52.9	1.06 (0.97–1.17)
No	63.2	64.4	1.00	13.4	8.5	1.00	47.6	51.4	1.00
Screened positive for depression									
Yes	60.5	63.6	1.04 (0.89–1.22)	21.4	9.5	1.14 (0.95–1.36)	61.8	55.6	1.21* (1.10–1.34)
No	62.0	62.7	1.00	12.0	8.4	1.00	46.2	50.9	1.00
Screened positive for generalized anxiety in past month									
Yes	61.4	63.8	1.05 (0.93–1.18)	25.4	10.9	1.35* (1.09–1.66)	67.1	58.1	1.34* (1.19–1.52)
No	61.8	62.8	1.00	12.2	8.3	1.00	46.6	50.9	1.00
Screened positive for PTSD in past month									
Yes	61.7	63.2	1.01 (0.83–1.24)	27.8	11.2	1.38* (1.12–1.69)	66.3	53.3	1.07 (0.90–1.26)
No	61.7	62.9	1.00	12.3	8.4	1.00	47.5	51.7	1.00
High work or family stress in past 12 months									
Yes	60.0	61.5	0.91* (0.84–0.99)	17.6	8.5	0.97 (0.85–1.11)	57.6	55.5	1.25* (1.16–1.36)
No	62.8	63.6	1.00	12.1	8.7	1.00	45.0	49.8	1.00
Active coping	–	–	0.98 (0.92–1.04)	–	–	1.02 (0.95–1.09)	–	–	1.07* (1.01–1.14)
Total	*61.8*	*61.8*	–	*14.3*	*14.3*	–	*49.5*	*49.5*	–
R²	–	–	*0.10*	–	–	*0.12*	–	–	*0.15*

Source: DoD Survey of Health Related Behaviors Among Active Duty Military Personnel, 2008

Note: Estimates are percentages among military personnel in each sociodemographic group that reported overweight/obese, illness, and injury.

*Odds ratio is significantly different from the reference group

[a]OR = Odds ratios were adjusted for all other independent variables in the model

[b]95 % CI = 95 % confidence interval of the odds ratio

(49.4 %) whereas senior enlisted personnel were the most likely to be overweight (70.4 %). The Navy had the highest likelihood of being overweight whereas the Marine Corps had the lowest. Personnel who had never deployed were significantly less likely to be overweight than those who had deployed.

Factors associated with a lower risk of overweight were high work or family stress, cigarette smoking, risk-taking, and high levels of spirituality.

4.3.2 Illness

Table 4.4 also shows the risk and protective factors for self-reported illness that kept service members from duty for a week or longer in the past 12 months. Women were significantly more likely than men to report having an illness in the past year, and whites were significantly less likely than African Americans to report an illness. Enlisted personnel, especially warrant officers, had a significantly greater risk of illness than senior officers. Combat exposure had a bimodal relationship with illness: both those with high combat exposure and those who had not deployed at all were more likely to report an illness compared to those who had been deployed but had no combat exposure.

By far the greatest risk factor for illness was having an injury in the past 12 months. Personnel reporting an injury had 7.5 times greater odds of an illness than those without an injury. Other significant risk factors were illicit drug use in the past month and screening positive for anxiety or posttraumatic stress disorder (PTSD). Factors associated with a significantly lower risk of illness included moderate or vigorous exercise and reporting moderate to low levels of spirituality compared to a high level of spirituality.

4.3.3 Injury

Table 4.4 also examines risk and protective factors for injury within the past year. As shown, women were more likely to report an injury than men, and younger personnel were at much lower risk for injury than older personnel. In contrast to the increased risk of illness among warrant officers, warrant officers were significantly *less* likely to report an injury than personnel in other pay grades. Service members in the Army and Marines were at higher risk for injury than those in the Navy and Air Force. Similar to the relationship between combat exposure and illness, those who had never deployed and those with moderate combat exposure were at the highest risk for injury.

Echoing the finding from the illness model, the greatest risk factor for injury was having an illness in the past 12 months. On the other hand, there were unique risk factors for injury not observed in the illness model, including having a history of physical or sexual abuse, getting an average of fewer than 7 h of nightly sleep, being overweight or obese, reporting high work or family stress, and screening positive for depression. In contrast with the illness model, those who reported a medium level of spirituality were at higher risk for an injury than those with high or low levels. Active coping was also a significant risk factor, which may be because participation in sports was included as a form of active coping. Similar to the illness model, illicit drug use in the past month and screening positive for anxiety were also risk factors for injury.

4.4 Summary and Discussion

4.4.1 Healthy People *Objectives*

Military service members met or exceeded two of the nine *Healthy People 2010* objectives that we examined: exercise and obesity. The seven objectives that were not met were cigarette use, smokeless tobacco use, binge drinking, illicit drug use, healthy weight, fruit intake, and vegetable intake. It is noteworthy that the exercise and obesity objectives that were met are those where the military has regulations that mandate minimal performance standards for these behaviors. Although progress has been made in improving the rates for some of the objectives that were not met, these efforts were still insufficient to reach the *Healthy People 2010* objectives. Clearly, more work is needed to reach the substance use, healthy weight, and healthy diet objectives. It may be challenging to reach these goals because many of these objectives will require service members to take some personal initiative for which they may not have the motivation or perhaps see the value.

4.4.2 *Overweight/Obesity*

Trend data for overweight/obesity showed a disturbing increase for the percentage of personnel having a BMI of 25 or higher from 50 % in 1995 to 60 % in 2008, which represents a 20 % increase over the 13-year period. Although this finding is consistent with the pattern of increasing overweight observed in the civilian population (Flegal et al., 2010), it was surprising to see it in the military in view of the heavy emphasis that the military places on physical fitness. This finding suggests that other factors, such as dietary intake or genetic factors, may play a role in overweight as suggested by Lindquist and Bray (2001). Regardless of the exact underlying factors accounting for overweight, one encouraging aspect of the trend data is that the rate of overweight/obesity for 2008 was nearly identical to the rate for 2005, suggesting a possible leveling off of the increase and hopefully a change in the trend line.

The results from the regression analyses showed that age, gender, and pay grade were the strongest predictors of overweight/obesity. After adjusting for all other variables in the model, personnel 20 or younger were 70 % less likely to be over-weight than those aged 35 or older; personnel aged 21–25 were 60 % less likely and personnel aged 26–34 were 30 % less likely to be overweight than those aged 35 or older. Overweight appeared to reach its peak at around age 35 in the active duty military population. The relationship of age to overweight is not surprising in that there is a tendency for personnel, even in the military, to become more involved in administrative responsibilities, which typically are more sedentary, as they become older. Indeed, our analyses indicated that although military personnel exercise more on average than civilians, the rates of vigorous exercise still declined significantly as service members got older. It is encouraging that the rate of overweight/obesity seemed to peak by about age 35 and did not increase further. Nonetheless, this remains a concern in that the rates of overweight/obesity peaked at a high level (nearly 75 %) by age 35.

Women were 62 % less likely to be overweight or obese than men. This was the case despite the fact that women were less likely than men to engage in vigorous exercise (55.7 % vs. 65.8 %). This finding suggests that women may have greater concern about weight, perhaps due to social influences, or perhaps may be more conscious of eating a healthier diet or controlling portion sizes to help manage their weight. Pay grade was also a strong predictor of overweight even after controlling for age and other related variables. Enlisted personnel and warrant officers were more likely to be overweight than commissioned officers. Senior enlisted personnel (E7–E9) were 2.4 times more likely to be overweight than senior officers and had the highest prevalence of overweight at 70 %. Because senior enlisted personnel tend to be the role models for more junior enlisted cadre, interventions aimed at helping them address issues of overweight may also have a trickle-down effect in helping them model improved fitness for other enlisted persons.

It is important to note that military personnel with BMIs within the overweight range are assumed to be overweight due to excess adiposity. Although BMI is a widely used and convenient measure of body composition, the term "overweight due to excess fat" may not be applicable to all military personnel. Muscled individu-als with an accumulation of lean body mass and a BMI of 25 or higher may be clas-sified as overweight even if their percent body fat is within a healthy range. Therefore, the military uses BMI and additional standards to confirm weight, including abdominal adiposity based on waist circumference, concomitant risk fac-tors for obesity-related chronic disease such as diabetes, and other techniques such as skin fold measurement and bioelectrical impedance (Kuczmarski & Flegal, 2000). Thus, although BMI has been adopted as the standard in civilian populations and is the most practical assessment for use in surveys, it is only one measure of body composition used by the military and may not be the best measure given the above limitations.

The findings that the military are far below the nutritional standards recom-mended by *Healthy People 2010*, in combination with the data on exercise and overweight, suggest that poor diet rather than a lack of exercise may play a critical role in the weight gain observed in the military.

4.4.3   Illness

Trends for illnesses showed a sharp reduction (by over half) from 1995 to 1998 followed by stable rates in 2002 and 2005 and then an increase in 2008. It is encouraging to see the reduction in illness rates in 1998, but it is unclear why the rates dropped so sharply. The increase in 2008 may be related to the increase in injuries. Although the illness rate increased in 2008, it was still well below the peak rate observed in 1995.

The results from the regression analyses showed that injury was the strongest predictor of illness. After adjusting for all other variables in the model, service members with an injury in the past year were 7.5 times more likely to report an illness than those without an injury. This is not surprising since injuries, especially more serious ones, can lead to shock and other physical illness symptoms; possible infections resulting from wound injuries; and variations in healing time based on the seriousness of the injury, how well the patient adheres to medical advice and directions, and the psychological perceptions of patients. In this latter regard, Wilson et al. (2011) found that respondents' attitudes and perceptions were positively associated with healing time from burn wounds.

Other important predictors of illness were military pay grade, combat exposure, gender, substance use and mental health variables, and exercise. Warrant officers were 2.4 times more likely, and enlisted personnel were from 1.5 to 1.9 times more likely than senior officers to report an illness in the past year that kept them from duty for a week or longer. These higher rates of illness among warrant officers and enlisted personnel may be associated with several factors such as type of work, work settings and work conditions, closeness of contact with associates, lifestyle habits such as hygiene practices, education of members, and overall general health and susceptibility to illness.

Those reporting high combat exposure were 1.6 times more likely to report an illness, and those who had not been deployed were 1.3 times more likely to report an illness compared to those to those who had been deployed but had no combat exposure. This bimodal relationship may reflect different environmental factors at play for these two groups. Those with high combat exposure may experience a more challenging physical environment (e.g., more dust or dirt) along with being at higher risk for both minor and major wounds and injuries (e.g., cuts, sprains, broken bones, combat-inflicted wounds) that may be associated with illnesses. In contrast, those who are not deployed are subject to the common illnesses present in the local civilian and military community, which may be higher than for those who are deployed but in a relatively safe setting where they have less exposure to family and community illnesses.

Military women were 1.7 times more likely than military men to report having an illness that kept them from duty for a week or longer. This is consistent with other studies that have shown higher rates of physical symptom reporting and health care utilization by women (Green & Pope, 1999; Kroenke & Spitzer, 1998). Similar to our findings, Kroenke and Spitzer (1998) found higher symptom reporting by women even after controlling for psychiatric comorbidity.

Personnel who used illicit drugs, who screened positive for anxiety, or who screened positive for PTSD were 35–45 % more likely to report illness than their counterparts. This suggests that personnel in these groups may be less diligent in caring for their health than their counterparts. Illicit drugs may lower the resistance of personnel making them more susceptible to illness. Anxiety and PTSD may lead service members to ignore good health practices, which in turn may result in greater illness.

Finally, analyses showed that persons who exercised regularly at moderate or vigorous levels were less likely to become ill than those who did not exercise at those levels. Personnel who engaged in regular exercise may be in better physical condition than their counterparts, which may permit them to avoid illness. Alternatively, those who exercised regularly may also have taken better care of themselves physically, including getting adequate sleep, eating more nutritious food, and perhaps practicing better hygiene such that they were better able to avoid illness.

4.4.4 Injury

Trend data showed that injury rates were relatively low—around 15 %—from 1995 to 2002, but then increased to 39 % in 2005 and remained at that level in 2008. The sharp increase in injury rates for 2005 and 2008 are most likely attributable to heightened tempo associated with training for combat or to war injuries from the conflicts in Iraq and Afghanistan. Clearly, service members engaged in combat were at much higher risk of injury, with most serious injuries resulting in death, as noted in Table 4.1, compared to those engaged in peace time activities.

As previously noted, illnesses are strongly related to injuries. This was further confirmed in our regression analyses, which showed that illness was the strongest predictor of injury. Service members with an illness that kept them from duty for at least a week in the past year were 7.5 times more likely to report an injury than those without such an illness. This follows when considering that the military population is generally young and in excellent health. Thus, when an illness occurs that lasts a week or more, it is often precipitated by an injury that requires a longer healing period. An analysis of injuries among nondeployed personnel found that injuries were the leading cause of medical encounters, with fractures being the most common type of injury requiring hospitalization, and sprains and strains being the most common type of injury resulting in outpatient visits (Jones, Canham-Chervak, Canada, Mitchener, & Moore, 2010).

Other strong predictors of injury were age, service, pay grade, history of physical or sexual abuse, reduced nightly sleep, illicit drug use, and anxiety. Age was positively related to injury risk. Persons aged 35 or older were twice as likely to have an injury as those aged 20 or younger. The finding that personnel in the Army (OR = 1.67) and Marine Corps (OR = 1.42) were at higher risk for injury is consistent with and most likely due to their combat-related missions. Active participation in the conflicts in Iraq and Afghanistan has placed these personnel at higher risk for injuries compared to personnel in the Air Force, who have been in more protected areas.

Military pay grade was also related to injury. In particular, warrant officers were the least likely of any pay grade group to experience an injury. This is likely related to their job activities. Warrant officers are technical specialists serving in positions that require the authority of an officer. However, in comparison with commissioned officers, warrant officers are heavily concentrated in engineering and maintenance occupations and, in some of the services, in intelligence and administrative positions.

Service members with a prior history of physical or sexual abuse were nearly 40 % more likely to report an injury than those who had not been abused. This is likely related to the fact that prior abuse is a key predictor of future abuse (Browne & Finkelhor, 1986; Farrington, 1991; Schumacher, Feldbau-Kohn, Smith, & Heyman, 2001; Stith, Smith, & Penn, 2004). Victims often adopt the role of victim, which may lead others to take advantage of their apparent weakness and put them at heightened risk for future abuse and injury.

Lack of sleep was another risk factor for injuries. Those who got 4 h or less of nightly sleep were 35 % more likely to report an injury in the past year. This is consistent with other research showing that sleep deprivation is related to accidents (Spengler, Browning, & Reed, 2004).

Personnel who screened positive for generalized anxiety disorder or who used illicit drugs were 34–39 % more likely to report injury than their counterparts. This is consistent with literature showing that antianxiety medications and illicit drugs impair cognitive functioning and result in loss of coordination and drowsiness, which in turn increase the risk of accidents, falls, and the like (Bolton et al., 2008).

4.5 Recap

Healthy and fit service members are critical to a ready and effective military force. Many factors affect the health of military personnel, including exposure to disease, risk of illness and injury in the performance of military duties, and lifestyle choices related to diet and nutrition, exercise, and substance use. A review of nine *Healthy People 2010* objectives indicated that the military met or exceeded the targets for two of them (exercise and obesity), but had not met the goals for the other seven (cigarette use, smokeless tobacco use, binge drinking, illicit drug use, healthy weight, fruit intake, and vegetable intake). The exercise and obesity objectives that were met are those where the military has regulations that mandate minimal performance standards for these behaviors. It may be challenging to meet the targets for the other objectives because they will require service members to take personal initiative for which they may not have the motivation or perhaps see the value.

Overweight/obesity trends showed a 20 % increase from 50 % in 1995 to 60 % in 2008, although the rate for 2008 was nearly identical to the rate for 2005, suggesting a possible leveling off of the increase. In view of the emphasis that the military places on physical fitness, the relatively high rates of exercise suggest that other factors, such as dietary intake or genetic indicators, likely play a critical role in the weight gain observed in the military. Age was the strongest predictor of overweight with personnel aged 20 or younger being nearly 70 % less likely to be overweight or obese than those 35 or older. There was a strong increase in the proportion of overweight or obese personnel with each advancing age group (ranging from 43.2 % to 73.8 %). Gender and pay grade were also strong predictors of overweight. Women were 62 % less likely to be overweight than men, and senior enlisted personnel were the most likely to be overweight across the pay grades (70.4 %).

Illness trends showed a sharp decrease from 1995 to 1998 followed by stable rates in 2002 and 2005 and then an increase in 2008. It is encouraging to see the reduction in 1998, but it is unclear why the rates dropped so sharply or why they increased in 2008, although the latter may be related to the increase observed in injuries during this same period. Indeed having an injury that kept persons from work for a week or longer was the strongest predictor of illness. Other important predictors of illness were military pay grade, combat exposure, gender, substance use and mental health variables, and exercise.

Injuries have been called the biggest health problem facing the military (Jones, Canham-Chervak, Canada, et al., 2010). Injury rates as measured by the HRB surveys were around 15 % from 1995 to 2002, but then increased to 39 % in 2005 and 2008; this increase is most likely attributable to injuries from heightened training for combat or to injuries from the conflicts in Iraq and Afghanistan. Illness was the strongest predictor of injury. Service members with an illness that kept them from duty for at least a week in the past year were 7.5 times more likely to report an injury than those without such an illness. Other important predictors of injury were being aged 35 or older, serving in the Army or Marine Corps, having a history of physical or sexual abuse, getting less than 7 h of nightly sleep, using illicit drugs, and screening positive for anxiety.

Maintaining good health and fitness for duty requires attention to a myriad of factors that span physical, emotional, and social domains.

References

Bolton, J. M., Metge, C., Lix, L., Prior, H., Sareen, J., & Leslie, W. D. (2008). Fracture risk from psychotropic medications: A population-based analysis. *Journal of Clinical Psychopharmacology, 28*, 384–391.

Bray, R. M., Hourani, L. L., Rae, K. L., Dever, J. A., Brown, J. M., Vincus, A. A., et al. (2006). *2002 Department of Defense survey of health related behaviors among military personnel*: *Final report* (prepared for the Assistant Secretary of Defense [Health Affairs], U.S. Department of Defense, Cooperative Agreement No. DAMD17-00-2-0057/RTI/7841/006-FR). Research Triangle Park, NC: Research Triangle Institute.

Bray, R. M., Hourani, L. L., Rae Olmsted, K. L., Witt, M., Brown, J. M., Pemberton, M. R., et al. (2006). *2005 Department of Defense survey of health related behaviors among active duty military personnel* Final report (prepared for the Assistant Secretary of Defense [Health Affairs], U.S. Department of Defense, Cooperative Agreement No. DAMD17-00-2-0057/RTI/7841/106-FR). Research Triangle Park, NC: Research Triangle Institute.

Bray, R. M., Kroutil, L. A., Wheeless, S. C., Marsden, M. E., Bailey, S. L., Fairbank, J. A., et al. (1995). *1995 Department of Defense survey of health related behaviors among military personnel* (DoD Contract No. DASO1-94-C-0140). Research Triangle Park, NC: Research Triangle Institute.

Bray, R. M., Pemberton, M. R., Hourani, L. L., Witt, M., Rae Olmsted, K. L., Brown, J. M., et al. (2009). *2008 Department of Defense survey of health related behaviors among active duty military personnel*. Report prepared for TRICARE Management Activity, Office of the Assistant Secretary of Defense (Health Affairs) and U.S. Coast Guard. Research Triangle Park, NC: Research Triangle Institute.

Bray, R. M., Pemberton, M., Lane, M. E., Hourani, L. L., Mattiko, M., & Babeu, L. A. (2010). Substance use and mental health trends among U.S. military active duty personnel: Key findings from the 2008 DoD Health Behavior Survey. *Military Medicine, 175*(6), 390–399.

Bray, R. M., Rae Olmsted, K. L., Williams, J., Sanchez, R. P., & Hartzell, M. (2006). Progress toward Healthy People 2000 objectives among U.S. military personnel. *Preventive Medicine, 42*(5), 390–396.

Bray, R. M., Sanchez, R. P., Ornstein, M. L., Lentine, D., Vincus, A. A., Baird, T. U., et al. (1999). *1998 Department of Defense survey of health related behaviors among military personnel: Final report* (prepared for the Assistant Secretary of Defense [Health Affairs], U.S. Department of Defense, Cooperative Agreement No. DAMD17-96-2-6021, RTI/7034/006-FR). Research Triangle Park, NC: Research Triangle Institute.

Browne, A., & Finkelhor, D. (1986). Impact of child sexual abuse: A review of the research. *Psychological Bulletin, 99,* 66–77.

Centers for Disease Control and Prevention. (2007). Prevalence of regular physical activity among adults—United States, 2001 and 2005. *Morbidity and Mortality Weekly Report, 56*(46), 1209–1212.

Crowe, A. H., & Bilchik, S. (1998). *Drug identification and testing summary*. Retrieved from http://www.ojjdp.gov/pubs/drugid/contents.html

Department of Defense. (1972). *Directive No. 1010.2. Alcohol abuse by personnel of the Department of Defense*. Washington, DC: U.S. Department of Defense.

Department of Defense. (1980a). *Directive No. 1010.4. Alcohol and drug abuse by DoD personnel*. Washington, DC: Deputy Secretary of Defense. Reissued September 3, 1997.

Department of Defense. (1980b). *Instruction No. 1010.5. Education and training in alcohol and drug abuse prevention*. Washington, DC: U.S. Department of Defense.

Department of Defense. (1985a). *Instruction No. 1010.6. Rehabilitation and referral services for alcohol and drug abusers*. Washington, DC: Author.

Department of Defense. (1985b). *Directive No. 1010.3. Drug and alcohol abuse reports* (cancelled by revised Directive 1010.4 on 3 Sept 1994; see DoD 1997). Washington, DC: Author.

Department of Defense. (1986). *Directive No. 1010.10. Health promotion*. Washington, DC: U.S. Department of Defense.

Department of Defense. (1997). *Directive No. 1010.4. Drug and alcohol abuse by DoD personnel*. Washington, DC: Author.

Department of Defense. (2003). *Directive No. 1010.10. Health promotion and disease/injury prevention*. Washington, DC: U.S. Department of Defense.

Department of Health and Human Services. (1996). *Physical activity and health: A report of the Surgeon General*. Atlanta, GA: U.S. Department of Health and Human Services, Centers for Disease Control and Prevention, National Center for Chronic Disease Prevention and Health Promotion.

Department of Health and Human Services. (2000). *Healthy People 2010: Understanding and improving health* (2nd ed.). Washington, DC: U.S. Government Printing Office.

Department of Health and Human Services. (2004). *The health consequences of smoking: A report of the Surgeon General*. Atlanta, GA: U.S. Department of Health and Human Services, Centers for Disease Control and Prevention, National Center for Chronic Disease Prevention and Health Promotion, Office on Smoking and Health.

Department of Health and Human Services/U.S. Department of Agriculture (DHHS/USDA). (2005). *Dietary guidelines for Americans*. Washington, DC: GPO.

Farrington, D. (1991). Childhood aggression and adult violence: Early precursors and later-life outcomes. In D. J. Pepler and K.H. Rubin (Ed.), *The development and treatment of childhood aggression* (pp. 5–29). New Jersey: Lawrence Erlbaum Associates, Inc.

Flegal, K. M. (2005). Estimating the impact of obesity. *Social and Preventive Medicine, 50*(2), 73–74.

Flegal, K. M., Carroll, M. D., Ogden, C. L., & Curtin, L. R. (2010). Prevalence and trends in obesity among U.S. adults, 1999–2008. *Journal of the American Medical Association, 303*(3), 235–241.

Green, C. A., & Pope, C. R. (1999). Gender psychosocial factors and the use of medical services: Longitudinal analyses. *Social Science & Medicine, 48*(10), 1363–1372.

Greenfield, L. A. (1998). *Alcohol and crime: An analysis of national data on the prevalence of alcohol involvement in crime*. Report prepared for the Assistant Attorney General's National Symposium on Alcohol Abuse and Crime. Washington, DC: U.S. Department of Justice.

Heron, M. (2012). Deaths: Leading causes for 2008. *National Vital Statistics Reports, 60*(6), 1–95.

Horgan, C., Skwara, K. C., & Strickler, G. (2001). *Substance abuse: The nation's number one health problem*. Princeton, NJ: The Robert Wood Johnson Foundation.

Institute of Medicine (IOM). (2010a). *Gulf war and health, Vol. 8: Update on health effects of serving in the Gulf War*. Washington, DC: National Academy Press.

Institute of Medicine (IOM). (2010b). *Veterans and Agent Orange: Update 2010*. Washington, DC: National Academy Press.

Jonas, W., Deuster, P., O'Conner, F., & Macedonia, C. (Eds.). (2010). Total force fitness for the 21st century: A new paradigm. *Supplement to Military Medicine, 175*, 8.

Jones, B. H., Amoroso, P. J., Canham, M. L., Weyandt, M. B., & Schmitt, J. B. (Eds.). (1999). Atlas of injuries in the U.S. armed forces. *Military Medicine, 164*(Suppl 8), S1–S633.

Jones, B. H., Canham-Chervak, M., Canada, S., Mitchener, T. A., & Moore, S. (2010). Medical surveillance of injuries in the U.S. Military: Descriptive epidemiology and recommendations for improvement. *American Journal of Preventive Medicine, 38*(1 Suppl), S42–S60.

Jones, B. H., Canham-Chervak, M., & Sleet, D. A. (2010). An evidence-based public health approach to injury priorities and prevention: Recommendations for the U.S. *Military American Journal of Preventive Medicine, 38*(1 Suppl), S1–S10.

Jones, B. H., & Hansen, B. C. (Eds.). (1996). *Injuries in the military: A hidden epidemic*. Report prepared by the Armed Forces Epidemiological Board Injury Prevention and Control Work Group. Report available from Defense Technical Information Center (DTIC) ADA322223.

Jones, B. H., Perrotta, D. M., Canham-Chervak, M. L., Nee, M. A., & Brundage, J. F. (2000). Injuries in the military: A review and commentary focused on prevention. *American Journal of Preventive Medicine, 18*(3 Suppl), 71–84.

Kaiser Family Foundation. (2002). *Substance use and risky sexual behavior: Attitudes and practices among adolescents and young adults*. Washington, DC: Author.

Knapik, J. J., Sharp, M. A., Darakjy, S., Jones, S. B., Hauret, K. G., & Jones, B. H. (2006). Temporal changes in the physical fitness of U.S. army recruits. *Sports Medicine, 36*(7), 613–634.

Kroenke, K., & Spitzer, R. L. (1998). Gender differences in the reporting of physical and somatoform symptoms. *Psychosomatic Medicine, 60*, 150–155.

Kuczmarski, R. J., & Flegal, K. M. (2000). Criteria for definition of overweight in transition: Background and recommendations for the United States. *American Journal of Clinical Nutrition, 72*, 1074–1081.

Lindquist, C. H., & Bray, R. M. (2001). Trends in overweight and physical activity among US military personnel, 1995–1998. *Preventive Medicine, 32*(1), 57–65.

McCluskey, C. P., Krohn, M. D., Lizotte, A. J., & Rodriguez, M. L. (2002). Early substance use and school achievement: An examination of Latino, White, and African American youth. *Journal of Drug Issues, 32*(3), 921–943.

McNulty, V. (2009). Injuries: The modern military epidemic. *Health tips from army medicine*. Retrieved April 1, 2010, from http://www.army.mil/article/25626/Injuries_the_modern_military_epidemic

Mokdad, A. H., Serdula, M. K., Dietz, W. H., Bowman, B. A., Marks, J. S., & Koplan, J. P. (1999). The spread of the obesity epidemic in the United States, 1991–1998. *Journal of the American Medical Association, 282*(16), 1519–1522.

National Center on Addiction and Substance Abuse at Columbia University. (1999). *No safe haven: Children of substance-abusing parents*. Retrieved April 1, 2010, from http://www.casa columbia.org/templates/publications_reports.aspx

National Center on Addiction and Substance Abuse at Columbia University. (2001). *Malign neglect: Substance abuse and America's schools*. New York, NY: Author.

Office of National Drug Control Policy. (2003). *Drug facts: Juveniles and drugs*. Retrieved March 29, 2010, from http://www.whitehousedrugpolicy.gov/drugfact/juveniles/

Office of the Assistant Secretary of Defense (Health Affairs). (1992). *Health status indicators for health promotion and disease prevention: Selected Healthy People 2000 objectives for the Department of Defense [Memorandum]*. Washington, DC: Author.

Office on Smoking and Health. (1989). *Reducing the health consequences of smoking: 25 years of progress: A report of the Surgeon General* (DHHS Publication No. CDC 89-8411). Washington, DC: U.S. Department of Health and Human Services.

Pinder, E., Gilbert, A., Rhodes, J., Brown, D., & Bates, M. (2011). *Worksite heath promotion: Wellness in the workplace*. Silver Spring, MD: Defense Centers of Excellence for Psychological Health and Traumatic Brain Injury.

Public Health Service. (1979). *Healthy people: The Surgeon General's report on health promotion and disease prevention* (DHEW Publication No. PHS 79-55071). Washington, DC: U.S. Department of Health, Education, and Welfare.

Public Health Service. (1980). *Promoting health/preventing disease: Objectives for the nation*. Washington, DC: U.S. Department of Health and Human Services.

Public Health Service. (1991). *Health people 2000: National health promotion and disease prevention objectives—Full report, with commentary* (DHHS Publication No. PHS 91-50212). Washington, DC: U.S. Department of Health and Human Services.

Robbins, A. S., Chao, S. Y., Russ, C. R., & Fonseca, V. P. (2002). Costs of excess body weight among active duty personnel, U.S. Air Force, 1997. *Military Medicine, 167*(5), 393–397.

Schumacher, J. A., Feldbau-Kohn, S., Smith, A. M., & Heyman, R. E. (2001). Risk factors for male-to-female partner physical abuse. *Aggression and Violent Behavior, 6*, 281–352.

Smith, G. S., Branas, C. C., & Miller, T. R. (1999). Fatal nontraffic injuries involving alcohol: A metaanalysis. *Annals of Emergency Medicine, 33*(6), 659–668.

Spengler, S. E., Browning, S. R., & Reed, D. B. (2004). Sleep deprivation and injuries in part-time Kentucky farmers: Impact of self-reported sleep habits and sleep problems on injury risk. *Journal of the American Association of Occupational Health Nurses, 52*(9), 373–382.

Stanley, J., & Blair, J. D. (Eds.). (1993). *Challenges in military health care: Perspectives on health status and the provision of care*. New Brunswick, NJ: Transaction Publishers.

Stith, S. M., Smith, D. B., & Penn, C. E. (2004). Intimate partner physical abuse perpetration and victimization risk factors: A meta-analytic review. *Aggression and Violent Behavior, 10*, 65–98.

Subcommittee of the President's Council on Fitness, Sports & Nutrition. (2012). *Physical activity guidelines for Americans midcourse report: Strategies to increase physical activity among youth*. Washington, DC: U.S. Department of Health and Human Services.

Trent, L. K., & Hurtado, S. L. (1998). Longitudinal trends and gender differences in physical fitness and lifestyle factors in career U.S. Navy personnel (1983–1994). *Military Medicine, 163*(6), 398–407.

Warber, J. P., Boquist, S. H., & Cline, A. D. (1997). Fruit and vegetables in the service member's diet: Data from military institutional feeding studies. *Military Medicine, 162*(7), 468–471.

Wechsler, H., Davenport, A., Dowdall, G. W., Moeykens, B., & Castillo, S. (1994). Health and behavioral consequences of binge drinking in college: A national survey of students at 140 campuses. *Journal of the American Medical Association, 272*(21), 1672–1677.

Williamson, D. A., Martin, P. D., Allen, H. R., Most, M. M., Alfonso, A. J., Thomas, V., et al. (2002). Changes in food intake and body weight associated with basic combat training. *Military Medicine, 167*(3), 248–253.

Wilson, J. J. (2000). *Juvenile justice bulletin: Co-occurrence of delinquency and other problem behaviors*. Washington, DC: U.S. Department of Justice Office of Juvenile Justice and Delinquency Prevention.

Wilson, E. R., Wisely, J. A., Wearden, A. J., Dunn, K. W., Edwars, J., & Tarrier, N. J. (2011). Do illness perceptions and mood predict healing time for burn wounds: A prospective, preliminary study. *Journal of Psychosomatic Research, 71*(5), 364–366.

Windle, M., & Mason, W. A. (2004). General and specific predictors of behavioral and emotional problems among adolescents. *Journal of Emotional and Behavioral Disorders, 12*(1), 49–62.

Yore, M. M., Bell, N. S., Senier, L., & Amoroso, P. J. (2000). Progress toward attainment of the Healthy People 2000 objectives in the U.S. Army: Measured by health risk appraisal results. *American Journal of Preventive Medicine, 19*(2), 87–93.

Chapter 5
Stress and Mental Health

5.1 Overview and Background

Mental health problems are a significant source of medical and occupational morbidity for military personnel. The psychological toll of war has been studied in American troops for well over a century. However, research attention has been cyclical, and major advances in our understanding of military psychology have been made during and following periods of conflict (see Jones & Wessely, 2005; Kennedy & McNeil, 2006; Levy & Sidel, 2009; Moore & Reger, 2007; Pols & Oak, 2007). Deep concern over large numbers of psychological casualties in military personnel returning from Afghanistan and Iraq during Operation Enduring Freedom (OEF) and Operation Iraqi Freedom (OIF) has led to renewed impetus to identify those at risk for serious mental health problems and treat those already suffering from negative mental health consequences (e.g., Adler, Bliese, & Castro, 2011; American Psychological Association, 2007; Burnam, Meredith, Tanielian, & Jaycox, 2009; DoD, 2007; Hoge et al., 2004; Litz, 2007; Marmar, 2009; Office of the Surgeon Multinational Force-Iraq, 2006; Safran et al., 2009; Seal et al., 2008). Consequently, researchers have amassed valuable information on the mental health issues of Army and Marine Corps personnel returning from ground combat duty (Dolan & Ender, 2008). However, personnel in the Navy and Air Force may also be at risk for mental health problems because they are exposed to similar operational stressors associated with frequent deployments, physical and mental work stressors, and fatigue.

To assess the experiences of stress and mental health status in the U.S. active duty force as a whole, it is necessary to include personnel from all services in population-based epidemiological studies. The services vary considerably in their sociodemographic composition, which must be taken into consideration when assessing the mental health status of military personnel. Results from population-based epidemiological studies such as those reported in this chapter are critical for identifying trends in mental health problems and health service utilization. Specifically, these data help provide for optimal resource allocation, identify risk and protective factors that may be utilized in outreach, referral, and prevention

R.M. Bray et al., *Understanding Military Workforce Productivity: Effects of Substance Abuse, Health, and Mental Health*, DOI 10.1007/978-0-387-78303-1_5,
© Springer Science+Business Media New York 2014

programming, and provide an assessment of the perceived need for and barriers to obtaining mental health treatment within the active force.

Major epidemiological studies utilizing population-based methods to assess prevalence rates and risk factors for mental health problems in the military have often limited their scope by focusing on personnel with hospitalizations or personnel in a single service (e.g., Booth-Kewley & Larson, 2005; Gunderson & Hourani, 2001a, 2001b, 2003; Hoge et al., 2002), high-risk populations such as combat personnel (Hoge et al., 2005; Riddle, Sandersa, Jones, & Webb, 2008), or on a single disorder such as posttraumatic stress disorder (PTSD) (Terhakopian, Sinaii, Engel, Schnurr, & Hoge, 2008; Wittchen, Gloster, Beesdo, Schönfeld, & Perkonigg, 2009), depression (Black et al., 2004; Warner et al., 2007), or suicide (Desai, Rosenheck, & Desai, 2008; Hourani, Yuan, & Bray, 2003).

Findings from these studies have varied greatly depending on population, type of disorder, and screening instrumentation. For example, in one study, Vietnam veterans had a reported lifetime PTSD prevalence of 31 % (Dohrenwend et al., 2006). For U.S. Gulf War-era veterans, 6.2 % of veterans were diagnosed with PTSD that developed during deployment, but only 1.8 % of Gulf War-era veterans reported symptoms that met criteria for PTSD 10 years later (Toomey et al., 2007). In another study, battle-injured U.S. soldiers had a reported prevalence rate of 12 % for PTSD and 9 % for depression 4 months following hospitalization (Grieger et al., 2006); and deployed soldiers and Marines had an estimated prevalence rate of 16–17 % for major depression, PTSD, or generalized anxiety disorder (GAD) 3–4 months after their return from Iraq (Hoge et al., 2004) and 19 % 1 year after return from deployment (Hoge, Auchterlonie, & Milliken, 2006). Although it is likely that prevalence rates for PTSD and other psychological disorders vary depending on experiences during deployment, there has been a lack of uniformity in the measurement of PTSD and other psychological disorders, which likely contributes to the large discrepancies in estimates across different investigators.

Similar to the variability reported in the prevalence of psychological disorders, the number of risk factors for negative psychological outcomes studied in military personnel has varied across study and type of disorder. For example, studies of general psychological well-being have identified the impact of separation and foreign residence (Burrell, Durand, & Castro, 2006), traumatic event exposure (Hourani et al., 2003; Martin, Rosen, Durant, Knudson, & Stretch, 2000), work stress (Hourani et al., 2006; Pflanz, 2001), and anticipation of combat (Rosen, Wright, Marlowe, Bartone, & Gifford, 1999) as risk factors. Studies have also cited adequate sleep (Dolan, Adler, Thomas, & Castro, 2005), social support, and unit cohesion as protective factors (Martin et al., 2000). Among risk factors for PTSD identified in military populations are duration of deployment (McFarlane, 2009), sustaining battle injuries (MacGregor et al., 2009), exposure to combat and repeated exposures to combat (Bolton, 2001), mismatch between expectations about duration of deployment and reality (Rona et al., 2008), high levels of physical problems (Grieger et al., 2006), prior (pre-deployment) exposure to traumatic events in childhood (Owens et al., 2009), duty in Iraq (Hoge et al., 2004), and severity of combat guilt (Henning & Frueh, 1997). Maguen, Suvak, and Litz (2006) provide an excellent overview of preservice, service, and post-service risk factors for PTSD among military veterans.

Additional risk factors for other psychological disorders have also been studied in military personnel. Risk factors for depression, anxiety, and suicidality overlap with those associated with PTSD—combat deployment and level of combat exposure (Wells et al., 2010) and low military rank—but may also include other demographic characteristics such as female gender, divorced or single marital status, family history of mental illness and alcohol abuse, high levels of stress, loneliness, life-change events, obesity, problematic interpersonal relations, and more emotion-oriented and less task-oriented coping (Kress, Peterson, & Hartzell, 2006; Ritchie, Keppler, & Rothberg, 2003; Williams, Bell, & Amorosa, 2002). In contrast, approach-based coping (Sharkansky et al., 2000) and military hardiness appear to be protective factors (Dolan & Adler, 2006).

A recent collection of articles addressed the nature, theory, and management of combat stress and combat stress injuries (Nash, 2007a). The authors were careful to point out that not only are military stressors "uniquely powerful and uniquely unrelenting" compared to civilian life but also they must be understood in the context of military culture, which can make it difficult to acknowledge one's own stress or seek professional help (Nash, 2007b, p. 29). Although several studies have noted the reluctance of military personnel to seek help for emotional or psychological problems (Britt et al., 2008; Britt, Greene-Shortridge, & Castro, 2007; Hoge et al., 2004; Langston & Gould, 2007; Pietrzak, Johnson, Goldstein, Malley, & Southwick, 2009; Warner, Appenzeller, Mullen, Warner, & Grieger, 2008), much remains to be learned about beliefs regarding the impact of help-seeking on a military career and attitudes and stigma toward personnel seeking help for psychological problems.

The Department of Defense (DoD) Surveys of Health Related Behaviors Among Active Duty Military Personnel (HRB surveys) have provided the first population-based mental health data on active duty military personnel in all DoD active duty service branches worldwide. To assess the impact of stressful experiences, beginning in 1988 the HRB survey series started to include questions related to the stress and mental health of active duty personnel with more recent surveys adding additional questions. As in previous surveys (Bray et al., 1988, 1992, 1995, 1999, 2003, 2006), the most recent HRB survey in 2008 (Bray et al., 2009) asked respondents to appraise their levels of stress experience attributed to work and to their intimate and family relationships. As they had since 1995, respondents were also asked to provide information on the perceived impact of work-related and personal or family-related stress experiences on their military performance and the methods they used to cope with feeling stressed. In the 2002 survey, new measures were included to support the 1999 DoD initiatives to control combat stress among service members and to expand DoD's suicide prevention program (Bray et al., 2003). To obtain baseline prevalence information, items were added on anxiety symptoms and suicidal ideation. New to the 2005 survey were standardized instruments to screen for symptoms potentially due to serious psychological distress and PTSD (see Chap. 2 for details on measures). Such screeners are not clinical assessments of these conditions, but may suggest the need for further evaluation. Finally, the use of, perceived need for, and perceived career damage associated with mental health counseling by service were assessed, as well as the relationship between perceived career damage and selected mental health measures. This chapter presents findings related to exposure to challenges eliciting work and family stress, the issues of mental health, coping strategies, and help-seeking.

5.2   Trends in Stress and Mental Health Among Military Personnel

5.2.1   Trends in Work and Family Stress

The challenges in demanding military environments may elicit significant experiences of stress (Nash, 2007a; Orasanu & Backer, 1996). Maladaptive stress reactions among military personnel have been associated with temperament and character profiles (Elsass, 2001), and both job satisfaction and personality characteristics have been found to be predictors of occupational stress in the military (Carbone & Cigrang, 2001). Psychosocial theories of stress generally recognize the importance of cognitive factors in developing and maintaining stress-related symptoms and problems in life functioning. For example, Folkman and Lazarus (1980, 1985) proposed a psychosocial model that emphasizes the important role that appraisal plays in developing and maintaining stress-related adjustment problems. Indeed, a number of experimental and applied studies have shown robust relationships between individuals' appraisal of the level of stress associated with specific life events and their capacity to function effectively (see Foa, Steketee, & Olasov Rothbaum, 1989). Most studies examining deployment stressors have been limited to selected combat troops and/or veteran groups (e.g., Hoge et al., 2004; Vogt, Pless, King, & King, 2005), although a few recent studies have examined stress on military families and veterans' interpersonal relationships outside the military (e.g., Warner, Appenzeller, Warner, & Grieger, 2009). The HRB surveys present a unique opportunity to assess the degree to which deployment, work, and interpersonal challenges were cited as main sources of stress in the general military population and to assess how these challenges have changed over time. Personnel were asked to separately appraise their stress levels attributed to work and family challenges, as well as the degree to which their experience of stress interfered with performance of their military jobs.

Figure 5.1 shows that since 1988 personnel have attributed higher levels of stress to work than to their personal lives. However, perceptions of both high work stress and high family stress have significantly declined across survey years from a high of 52 % of personnel reporting high levels of work stress in 1992 to a low of 27 % in 2008. Although recent decreases in estimated levels of work stress were observed from 2005 to 2008, estimated levels of high family stress were mostly consistent between 2005 and 2008. Similar to the decline in reported work stress across survey years, high levels of family stress peaked at 33 % in 1992 before decreasing to a low of 18 % in 2008.

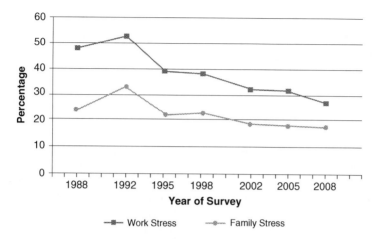

Fig. 5.1 Trends in high work and family stress among DoD personnel, 1988–2008

The rate for work stress in the total DoD services in 2008 (27.1 %) is similar to the estimated 26 % of work stress reported for a small group of personnel on an Air Force base (Pflanz & Sonnek, 2002), which is surprising since Air Force rates are generally lower than overall rates for DoD. The high stress rate observed by Pflanz and Sonnek (2002) is likely due to specific pressures experienced in their Air Force location, but from a sample that is not representative of the Air Force overall. In the 2008 HRB survey, which is population-based, Air Force personnel reported the lowest levels of work stress compared to Army, Navy, and Marine Corps personnel who generally have higher rates of combat exposure. This pattern of reporting was also observed in the 2005 HRB survey.

The overall declining trend in work stress noted in Fig. 5.1 initially appears counterintuitive during a period of war. This pattern is consistent, however, with the stages of adaptation model of perceived stress in combat and other military operations described by Nash (2007b) in which lower rates of perceived stress are indicative of "being in the groove" to adapt to the challenges of combat. In this model, it may be expected that rates would again increase postwar reflecting a "rebound" stress as service members "emerge from their emotional and physical numbness" (Nash, 2007b, p. 47). Despite these decreased rates, it should be noted that in 2008 28 % of all DoD personnel reported the experience of stress attributed to work interfered "some" or "a lot" with the performance of their military job, and 15 % reported that the experience of stress attributed to family issues interfered with their job performance more than "a little."

5.2.2   Specific Life Events to Which Stress Is Attributed

The last few HRB surveys have included specific questions in the domains of work and family life to enhance the understanding of perceived sources of stress among military personnel. Respondents were asked how much stress they experienced during the past 12 months in each of the domains listed in Table 5.1.

As shown in Table 5.1, the most frequently reported sources of stress for all DoD personnel in 2008 were being away from family, deployment, and increases in work load. Conflict between military and family responsibilities was the next most frequently reported source of stress, followed by permanent change of station (PCS) and problems with coworkers. These top sources of stress were reported by both genders, although several significant differences between men and women were observed. Women reported significantly more stress than men due to problems with supervisors or coworkers. Women also reported significantly more stress than men due to family concerns, such as finding childcare/daycare and divorce or breakup. Women also reported personal health problems as a greater source of stress compared to their male counterparts. On the other hand, a greater percentage of men reported high levels of stress because of deployment.

As shown in Table 5.1, in 2008, military personnel attributed their sources of highest stress to an increased number of stressful life events. Compared to both 2002 and 2005, military personnel in 2008 reported experiencing significantly increased stress related to having a PCS, being away from family, personal health problems, family health problems, and behavior problems in children. Compared to 2005, military personnel in 2008 reported experiencing significantly more stress related to the following life events: concern about performance rating, increases in work load, decreases in work load, insufficient training, finding childcare/daycare, death in the family, divorce or breakup, conflicts between military and family responsibilities, and problems with housing. When comparing data from 2008 to 2002 only, military personnel reported experiencing significantly more stress related to deployment. The pattern of results shows that both military men and women are attributing more stress to an increased number of stressful life events in the most recent 2008 survey compared to previous surveys in 2002 and 2005.

5.2.3 Coping with Stress

Respondents were asked to identify the types of strategies they used to cope when they "feel pressured, stressed, depressed, or anxious." The list of response categories included items that reflect active coping strategies (e.g., "think of plan to solve problem," "talk to friend or family member".) and avoidance coping strategies (e.g., "have a drink," "smoke marijuana or use other illegal drugs," "think about hurting yourself or killing yourself"). Table 5.2 shows the percentage of personnel, by gender and for the total DoD in 2008, who commonly used specific coping strategies under conditions of stress.

Overall, military personnel were more likely to use more constructive active coping strategies than avoidance coping strategies. When the responses of the total DoD were rank-ordered, each of the five active coping options was reported by more personnel than any of the five avoidance coping options. "Think of plan to

Table 5.1 Life events to which stress is attributed, past 12 months, by gender and year, 2002, 2005, and 2008, DoD personnel

Stressor	Men			Women			Total		
	2002	2005	2008	2002	2005	2008	2002	2005	2008
Deployment	12.3 (1.4)[a]	13.9 (1.2)	16.9 (1.5)[b]	8.8 (1.8)	10.1 (1.3)	13.1 (1.5)	11.7 (1.4)[a]	13.4 (1.2)	16.4 (1.4)[b]
Having a permanent change of station	5.3 (0.3)[a]	6.3 (0.8)[a]	9.5 (0.5)[b,c]	6.1 (0.5)[a]	6.4 (0.5)[a]	9.5 (0.8)[b,c]	5.5 (0.3)[a]	6.3 (0.7)[a]	9.5 (0.4)[b,c]
Problems with coworkers	9.4 (0.6)	8.1 (0.7)	8.8 (0.5)	13.5 (1.1)	11.8 (0.7)	12.8 (0.6)	10.1 (0.6)	8.6 (0.6)	9.4 (0.4)
Problems with supervisor	10.0 (0.7)	9.0 (0.7)	8.7 (0.4)	12.5 (0.7)	12.5 (0.8)	12.1 (0.6)	10.4 (0.6)	9.6 (0.7)	9.2 (0.4)
Concern about performance rating	5.6 (0.4)	5.0 (0.3)[a]	6.3 (0.2)[c]	5.6 (0.4)	6.6 (0.6)	6.9 (0.6)	5.6 (0.4)	5.2 (0.3)[a]	6.4 (0.2)[c]
Increases in work load	13.9 (0.8)	12.8 (0.5)[a]	14.7 (0.4)[c]	15.8 (0.8)	13.5 (0.8)[a]	15.9 (0.7)[c]	14.2 (0.7)	12.9 (0.5)[a]	14.9 (0.4)[c]
Decreases in work load	1.9 (0.2)[a]	1.7 (0.2)[a]	2.5 (0.2)[b,c]	2.9 (0.4)[a,c]	1.4 (0.2)[b]	1.9 (0.2)[b]	2.1 (0.2)	1.6 (0.2)[a]	2.4 (0.2)[c]
Insufficient training	NA NA	6.7 (0.4)[a]	8.8 (0.4)[c]	NA NA	8.1 (0.8)[a]	10.8 (0.8)[c]	NA NA	6.9 (0.4)[a]	9.1 (0.4)[c]
Being away from family	16.9 (1.0)[a]	16.6 (1.1)[a]	22.1 (1.2)[b,c]	18.6 (1.4)[a]	16.9 (1.0)[a]	24.7 (0.9)[b,c]	17.2 (1.0)[a]	16.6 (1.1)[a]	22.5 (1.1)[b,c]
Having a baby	NA NA	5.0 (0.4)[a]	6.6 (0.4)[c]	NA NA	6.8 (0.7)	8.1 (0.6)	NA NA	5.2 (0.3)[a]	6.8 (0.4)[c]
Finding childcare/daycare	NA NA	2.9 (0.2)[a]	4.8 (0.2)[c]	NA NA	7.3 (0.7)	9.0 (0.6)	NA NA	3.5 (0.2)[a]	5.4 (0.2)[c]
Death in family	NA NA	5.2 (0.3)[a]	6.5 (0.4)[c]	NA NA	6.7 (0.6)	7.9 (0.5)	NA NA	5.4 (0.3)[a]	6.7 (0.4)[c]
Divorce or breakup	NA NA	5.2 (0.4)[a]	7.3 (0.4)[c]	NA NA	9.0 (0.8)	9.4 (0.4)	NA NA	5.8 (0.4)[a]	7.6 (0.4)[c]
Infidelity or unfaithfulness by you or partner	NA NA	NA NA	6.3 (0.4)	NA NA	NA NA	8.7 (0.4)	NA NA	NA NA	6.7 (0.4)
Conflicts between military and family responsibilities	10.5 (0.6)[a]	9.0 (0.6)[a]	12.2 (0.6)[b,c]	13.0 (0.9)[c]	10.0 (0.8)[b]	11.8 (0.5)	10.9 (0.6)[a]	9.2 (0.5)[a,b]	12.2 (0.5)[c]
Problems with money	9.6 (0.7)	8.0 (0.6)	8.6 (0.5)	10.7 (0.8)[a,c]	7.5 (0.7)[b]	8.7 (0.4)[b]	9.8 (0.6)[c]	7.9 (0.6)[b]	8.6 (0.4)
Problems with housing	5.4 (0.3)[a,c]	4.2 (0.4)[a,b]	6.3 (0.3)[b,c]	5.8 (0.6)	5.2 (0.5)	5.7 (0.4)	5.4 (0.3)[c]	4.4 (0.3)[a,b]	6.2 (0.3)[c]
Personal health problems	3.6 (0.3)[a]	4.0 (0.4)[a]	5.7 (0.4)[b,c]	7.8 (0.5)	6.8 (0.9)	8.2 (0.4)	4.3 (0.3)[a]	4.4 (0.4)[a]	6.1 (0.4)[b,c]
Family health problems	5.6 (0.2)[a]	5.9 (0.4)[a]	6.9 (0.3)[b,c]	7.0 (0.7)	6.9 (0.6)	8.3 (0.4)	5.8 (0.2)[a]	6.0 (0.3)[a]	7.1 (0.3)[b,c]
Behavior problems in children	2.1 (0.2)[a]	2.1 (0.1)[a]	3.4 (0.2)[b,c]	3.3 (0.3)	2.9 (0.4)	3.7 (0.4)	2.3 (0.2)[a]	2.2 (0.1)[a]	3.4 (0.1)[b,c]
Unexpected event/problem	NA NA	3.1 (0.4)	3.1 (0.2)	NA NA	3.5 (0.6)	3.1 (0.2)	NA NA	3.1 (0.4)	3.1 (0.2)

Source: DoD Survey of Health Related Behaviors Among Active Duty Military Personnel, 2002, 2005, and 2008

Note: Table displays the percentage of military personnel reporting "a lot" of stress to the noted life events. The standard error of each estimate is presented in parentheses.

[a]Indicates estimate is significantly different from the estimate in column #3 (2008) at the 95 % confidence level

[b]Indicates estimate is significantly different from the estimate in column #1 (2002) at the 95 % confidence level

[c]Indicates estimate is significantly different from the estimate in column #2 (2005) at the 95 % confidence level

NA not applicable or data not available

Table 5.2 Behaviors for coping with stress, by gender, 2008

| | Gender | | |
Coping behavior	Men	Women	Total
Talk to friend/family member	71.3 (0.6)[a]	85.8 (0.6)[b]	73.4 (0.6)
Light up a cigarette	28.6 (1.0)[a]	21.0 (1.3)[b]	27.5 (1.0)
Have a drink	34.5 (1.0)[a]	25.2 (1.1)[b]	33.1 (1.0)
Say a prayer	46.7 (0.7)[a]	67.6 (1.7)[b]	49.7 (0.9)
Exercise or play sports	63.1 (0.8)	63.5 (1.4)	63.2 (0.8)
Engage in a hobby	64.3 (0.4)[a]	58.6 (1.1)[b]	63.4 (0.4)
Get something to eat	45.7 (0.7)[a]	56.2 (0.9)[b]	47.3 (0.6)
Smoke marijuana/use other illegal drugs	2.7 (0.3)[a]	1.2 (0.3)[b]	2.5 (0.2)
Think of plan to solve problem	78.5 (0.7)[a]	83.6 (0.7)[b]	79.3 (0.7)
Think about hurting or killing myself	5.1 (0.3)	4.9 (0.4)	5.1 (0.3)

Source: DoD Survey of Health Related Behaviors Among Active Duty Military Personnel, 2008
Note: Table displays the percentage of military personnel by gender who "frequently" or "sometimes" engaged in the indicated coping behavior when they felt pressured, stressed, depressed, or anxious. The standard error of each estimate is presented in parentheses.
[a]Indicates estimate is significantly different from the estimate in column #2 (women) at the 95 % confidence level
[b]Indicates estimate is significantly different from the estimate in column #1 (men) at the 95 % confidence level

solve problem" was overwhelmingly indicated by military personnel as a "frequently" or "sometimes" implemented coping strategy, followed by "talk to friend or family member," "engage in a hobby," "exercise or play sports," and "say a prayer." A solid majority of personnel often used these potentially active coping strategies to deal with stress, daily pressures, and feelings of depression. With respect to the generally less-effective avoidance coping strategies, 47.3 % of DoD personnel indicated that they "get something to eat" when confronted with stress, 33.1 % "have a drink," 27.5 % "light up a cigarette," 5.1 % consider hurting or killing themselves, and 2.5 % smoke marijuana or use other illegal drugs.

There were also significant gender differences in coping strategies. Women were more likely than men to report using social support, saying a prayer, thinking of a plan to solve the problem, or eating to cope with stress. In contrast, men were more likely than women to engage in hobbies or use alcohol, cigarettes, or illegal drugs as methods of coping. Both men and women were equally likely to exercise or play sports and consider self-harm as a coping mechanism.

5.2.4 Trends in Depression, Suicidal Thoughts When Stressed, and Receipt of Counseling

In the mid-1990s, the HRB surveys began incorporating indices of mental health to help assess the impact of occupational stressors. Initial measures included a screening

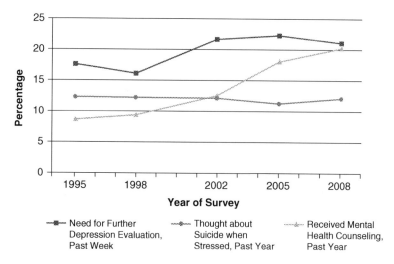

Fig. 5.2 Trends in mental health indicators among DoD personnel, 1995–2008

measure for depressive symptoms, a measure of suicidal ideation in response to stressors, and a measure of receipt of mental health counseling (see Chap. 2).

Figure 5.2 shows the percentages of military personnel who met the composite depression screening criterion across the past 5 survey years.

As shown in Fig. 5.2, the percentage of personnel meeting screening criteria for needing further depression evaluation increased from 1998 to 2005 and remained about the same in 2008. The sharpest increase occurred between 1998 with a low of 16.11 % and 2002 with a high of 22.31 %.

An increase was also seen among those who reported receiving mental health counseling during the same time period. These results depicted a more dramatic upward trend over the past five HRB surveys, with the highest percentage of personnel receiving counseling in 2008. The rates of personnel receiving counseling ranged from 9 % in 1995 to 20 % in 2008.

In contrast to the upward trend in depression symptoms and receipt of mental health counseling shown, there has been no significant difference across survey years in the percentage of personnel who reported thinking about suicide when feeling "pressured, stressed, depressed, or anxious." This estimated rate, which was 11.7 % in 2008, has remained steady between 11 and 12 % in every HRB survey since 1995. It should be noted that the percentage of DoD personnel who reported considering suicide when stressed is similar to the percentage of completed suicides in the military between 1996 (13.3 %) and 2002 (10.8 %), which generally approximates that of the total civilian population (Jones, Kennedy, & Hourani, 2006). This measure is also different from the measure of self-reported suicidal ideation in Sect. 5.3.

Because depression has long been associated with gender difference (with women having higher rates), we examined the rates of depression symptoms by service, gender, and year (data not shown). Although women's rates were higher than men's across all services and survey years, there was a significant increase in

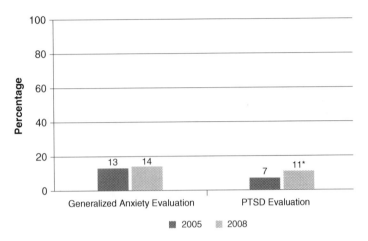

Fig. 5.3 Need for further evaluation of generalized anxiety and PTSD in past month among DoD personnel, 2005 and 2008
*Estimate is statistically significant from the 2005 estimate at the .05 level

personnel meeting screening criteria for depression among men in the Army and Marine Corps between 2002 and 2008 that was not reflected among their female counterparts.

5.2.5 Trends in Generalized Anxiety Disorder and Posttraumatic Stress Disorder

With the advent of the conflicts in Iraq and Afghanistan, the HRB surveys incorporated additional mental health screening instruments for GAD and PTSD symptoms (see Chap. 2 for a description of instruments). As shown in Fig. 5.3, the unadjusted current prevalence rates for GAD increased only slightly and not significantly between 2005 and 2008. An estimated 13 % in 2005 and 14 % in 2008 met screening criteria suggesting the need for further GAD evaluation. In contrast, the prevalence of PTSD increased 64 % from 2005 to 2008. That is, an estimated 7 % of the active force met screening criteria for PTSD in 2005, and this number rose to 11 % in 2008, indicating a large increase in the need for further PTSD evaluation during this period.

5.3 Correlates and Predictors of Mental Health Problems

To identify those personnel who may be at higher risk for negative mental health outcomes and to estimate the disease burden in population subgroups, the HRB surveys examined a large number of potential risk and protective factors for high work or family stress and for multiple mental health indicators. Following the conceptual model described in Chap. 1, Tables 5.3 and 5.4 show the prevalence and risk factors examined for high levels of stress and mental health outcomes based on multivariate logistic regression models conducted with the active duty survey data from 2008. Risk and protective factors that were not associated with any of the outcomes at the bivariate level, such as weight, were excluded from the models. Overall, the variables remaining in the models accounted for between 27 % of the variance in the depression indicator model and 7 % of the variance in the suicidal ideation indicator model.

5.3.1   Work and Family Stress

As shown in Table 5.3, 35.7 % of military personnel reported high levels of work or family stress. Unadjusted prevalence rates indicate that 62.7–73.0 % of those meeting screening criteria for a mental health problem—from depression symptoms to generalized anxiety—reported high stress compared to 34.3–27.2 % of those without such problems. After controlling for all variables in the logistic regression model, depression and generalized anxiety remained as the strongest predictors of high work or family stress. Those screening positive for these two problems were approximately 2.5 times more likely to report high work or family stress than their counterparts who did not screen positive. Other significant risk factors for high work or family stress were getting an average of less than 7 h of nightly sleep, avoidance coping, having a history of physical or sexual abuse, screening positive for PTSD, having an injury in the past 12 months, being a woman, being white, and being in the Navy. Protective factors were being enlisted and not being deployed.

5.3.2   Depression

As shown in Table 5.3, meeting screening criteria for further depression evaluation is associated with a number of sociodemographic and behavioral risk and protective factors. Consistent with findings on depression from major epidemiological surveys of psychiatric disorders in the U.S. civilian population, such as the Epidemiologic Catchment Area Study (Regier et al., 1990) and the National Comorbidity Survey (Kessler et al., 1994), the HRB surveys have found that a higher percentage of women than men respond to the depression screening questions by endorsing symptoms consistent with depression and consequently indicating a need for more comprehensive evaluation for depression. In 2008, the unadjusted percentage of women who had a score suggestive of a need for further depression evaluation was 25.7 % for the entire DoD. For men in the total DoD, 20.4 % screened positive for needing further depression evaluation.

Table 5.3 Correlates of stress, depression, and generalized anxiety, 2008

Independent variables	High work or family stress			Current depression			Generalized anxiety in past month		
	Unadjusted %	Adjusted %	Adjusted ORs[a] (95 % CI)[b]	Unadjusted %	Adjusted %	Adjusted ORs[a] (95 % CI)[b]	Unadjusted %	Adjusted %	Adjusted ORs[a] (95 % CI)[b]
Gender									
Male	34.7	34.4	1.00	20.4	15.1	1.00	13.3	6.8	1.00
Female	41.2	40.7	1.31* (1.18–1.45)	25.7	18.1	1.24* (1.08–1.43)	19.3	11.1	1.73* (1.43–2.09)
Age									
20 or younger	35.4	37.9	1.25 (0.99–1.57)	26.4	13.4	0.69* (0.52–0.91)	17.1	9.0	1.14 (0.68–1.92)
21–25	38.8	35.6	1.12 (0.91–1.38)	24.5	14.6	0.77* (0.66–0.89)	16.5	6.8	0.85 (0.61–1.19)
26–34	36.1	35.9	1.14 (0.94–1.38)	19.3	15.1	0.79* (0.66–0.95)	12.7	6.6	0.82 (0.62–1.10)
35 or older	31.2	32.9	1.00	15.9	18.3	1.00	11.2	7.9	1.00
Race/ethnicity									
White non-Hispanic	36.8	36.5	1.26* (1.12–1.42)	21.3	15.6	1.10 (0.93–1.31)	14.7	7.7	1.36* (1.11–1.67)
African American non-Hispanic	30.9	31.3	1.00	18.0	14.4	1.00	11.3	5.8	1.00
Hispanic	35.2	33.4	1.10 (0.93–1.31)	22.9	15.5	1.10 (0.89–1.35)	14.5	7.4	1.31 (0.94–1.84)
Other	36.7	34.0	1.14 (0.97–1.33)	24.3	16.3	1.16 (0.94–1.45)	15.3	6.2	1.08 (0.81–1.44)
Family status									
Not married	36.8	35.0	0.99 (0.87–1.12)	25.2	17.0	1.30* (1.16–1.47)	15.2	6.8	0.87 (0.75–1.01)
Married–spouse not present	39.2	36.5	1.06 (0.84–1.32)	25.1	19.1	1.50* (1.22–1.84)	15.2	6.8	0.88 (0.71–1.09)
Married–spouse present	33.8	35.3	1.00	16.6	13.6	1.00	12.9	7.7	1.00
Children living with you									
Yes	35.1	36.3	1.08 (0.95–1.23)	17.8	14.1	0.83* (0.74–0.93)	13.8	7.5	1.06 (0.87–1.30)
No	36.1	34.5	1.00	23.3	16.4	1.00	14.4	7.1	1.00

Pay grade								
E1–E3	35.1	32.1	0.65* (0.52–0.82)	27.0	16.5	1.10 (0.79–1.55)	16.8	6.8	1.17 (0.70–1.93)
E4–E6	38.3	34.9	0.73* (0.58–0.93)	22.8	15.5	1.03 (0.76–1.39)	15.8	7.7	1.33 (0.93–1.90)
E7–E9	29.3	32.6	0.66* (0.50–0.89)	14.8	13.6	0.88 (0.63–1.24)	11.2	7.6	1.31 (0.91–1.89)
W1–W5	25.4	31.2	0.62* (0.43–0.90)	14.4	14.8	0.97 (0.61–1.54)	7.2	5.9	0.99 (0.41–2.39)
O1–O3	33.2	40.4	0.93 (0.71–1.21)	13.7	15.9	1.06 (0.73–1.53)	8.1	6.4	1.08 (0.74–1.59)
O4–O10	32.5	42.2	1.00	12.8	15.2	1.00	7.9	5.9	1.00
Service								
Army	37.7	34.4	1.02 (0.91–1.15)	23.7	15.1	1.12 (1.00–1.27)	17.1	7.4	1.08 (0.90–1.28)
Navy	37.9	38.3	1.21* (1.06–1.39)	21.9	17.2	1.31* (1.07–1.60)	13.0	6.6	0.95 (0.74–1.23)
Marine Corps	37.8	34.9	1.05 (0.90–1.23)	25.9	17.0	1.29* (1.16–1.44)	17.3	8.3	1.21 (1.00–1.46)
Air Force	29.1	33.8	1.00	13.8	13.7	1.00	8.9	6.9	1.00
Deployment and combat exposure								
Not deployed	31.1	31.7	0.80* (0.69–0.93)	21.5	16.3	1.06 (0.88–1.27)	13.6	7.3	1.16 (0.91–1.48)
Deployed–none	33.1	36.0	1.00	17.4	15.6	1.00	10.1	6.4	1.00
Deployed–moderate	34.5	36.2	1.01 (0.87–1.17)	17.7	15.0	0.96 (0.81–1.13)	11.9	7.8	1.23* (1.01–1.52)
Deployed–high	42.9	38.2	1.10 (0.95–1.27)	26.3	14.9	0.95 (0.79–1.15)	20.4	7.5	1.19 (0.98–1.43)
Average hours of nightly sleep								
7+h	24.3	29.5	1.00	11.3	12.0	1.00	5.3	4.2	1.00
5–6 h	35.8	36.4	1.37* (1.19–1.59)	19.8	16.0	1.39* (1.19–1.62)	12.3	7.4	1.81* (1.50–2.19)
4 h or less	52.7	40.1	1.60* (1.27–2.01)	41.1	20.0	1.83* (1.54–2.19)	34.8	14.6	3.89* (3.07–4.92)
History of physical/sexual abuse								
Yes	45.8	40.3	1.46* (1.34–1.61)	30.5	18.8	1.52* (1.33–1.73)	21.0	7.9	1.20* (1.07–1.35)
No	28.4	31.5	1.00	14.5	13.2	1.00	9.2	6.7	1.00
Risk-taking/impulsivity								
High	51.7	37.9	1.14 (0.91–1.41)	39.7	17.1	1.14 (0.94–1.38)	31.4	9.5	1.38* (1.10–1.74)
Medium/low	34.1	35.0	1.00	19.4	15.3	1.00	12.5	7.0	1.00

(continued)

Table 5.3 (continued)

Independent variables	High work or family stress			Current depression			Generalized anxiety in past month		
	Unadjusted %	Adjusted %	Adjusted ORs[a] (95 % CI)[b]	Unadjusted %	Adjusted %	Adjusted ORs[a] (95 % CI)[b]	Unadjusted %	Adjusted %	Adjusted ORs[a] (95 % CI)[b]
Spirituality									
High	34.3	35.8	1.00	17.6	15.9	1.00	12.3	7.0	1.00
Medium	35.2	34.6	0.95 (0.85–1.07)	21.9	16.1	1.01 (0.85–1.21)	14.2	7.2	1.03 (0.82–1.29)
Low	37.0	35.9	1.01 (0.86–1.17)	22.8	14.2	0.87 (0.73–1.05)	15.3	7.4	1.05 (0.85–1.29)
Moderate/vigorous physical exercise in past month									
Yes	35.4	35.0	0.93 (0.82–1.06)	20.6	15.5	1.04 (0.87–1.24)	13.7	7.0	0.80* (0.66–0.97)
No	37.3	36.6	1.00	23.9	15.0	1.00	16.2	8.6	1.00
Illness in past 12 months									
Yes	44.5	34.5	0.96 (0.84–1.10)	32.4	16.9	1.13 (0.93–1.37)	25.7	9.1	1.33* (1.10–1.60)
No	34.2	35.4	1.00	19.4	15.3	1.00	12.3	7.0	1.00
Injury in past 12 months									
Yes	41.5	37.7	1.23* (1.14–1.34)	26.4	17.2	1.29* (1.12–1.48)	19.2	8.2	1.31* (1.13–1.52)
No	30.0	32.9	1.00	16.0	13.9	1.00	9.2	6.4	1.00
Illicit drug use in past month									
Yes	44.5	34.7	0.98 (0.87–1.10)	33.8	14.7	0.93 (0.74–1.18)	24.7	7.4	1.04 (0.80–1.33)
No	34.5	35.3	1.00	19.5	15.6	1.00	12.7	7.2	1.00
Risk for alcohol-related problems									
High risk (AUDIT 8+)	45.0	36.9	1.11 (1.00–1.24)	31.4	14.6	0.91 (0.74–1.11)	21.5	7.4	1.03 (0.84–1.26)
Low risk (AUDIT <8)	33.1	34.5	1.00	17.5	15.9	1.00	11.2	7.2	1.00
Screened positive for depression									
Yes	67.1	53.2	2.56* (2.32–2.83)	–	–	–	43.4	18.0	3.74* (3.28–4.27)
No	27.2	30.8	1.00	–	–	–	6.3	5.5	1.00

	%	%	OR (95% CI)	%	%	OR (95% CI)	%	%	OR (95% CI)
Screened positive for generalized anxiety in past month									
Yes	73.0	53.5	2.40* (2.07–2.78)	65.0	35.5	3.61* (3.14–4.15)	—	—	—
No	29.5	32.4	1.00	13.9	13.2	1.00	—	—	—
Screened positive for PTSD in past month									
Yes	72.5	43.2	1.46* (1.23–1.73)	74.5	38.8	4.03* (3.31–4.91)	63.3	26.8	5.67* (4.84–6.64)
No	31.2	34.3	1.00	14.8	13.6	1.00	8.3	6.1	1.00
High work or family stress in past 12 months									
Yes	—	—	—	39.9	25.3	2.64* (2.39–2.91)	29.0	12.4	2.56* (2.19–2.98)
No	—	—	—	10.8	11.4	1.00	5.9	5.2	1.00
Suicidal ideation in past 12 months									
Yes	62.7	42.2	1.36 (1.00–1.85)	62.8	39.4	3.78* (2.95–4.86)	40.4	7.5	1.05 (0.79–1.40)
No	34.3	34.9	1.00	19.2	14.7	1.00	12.9	7.2	1.00
Active coping	—	—	1.11 (1.00–1.22)	—	—	0.73* (0.67–0.80)	—	—	1.03 (0.88–1.19)
Avoidance coping	—	—	1.54* (1.37–1.74)	—	—	2.22* (1.93–2.57)	—	—	1.45* (1.23–1.71)
Total	35.7	35.7	—	21.2	21.2	—	14.2	14.2	—
R^2	—	—	0.17	—	—	0.27	—	—	0.25

Source: DoD Survey of Health Related Behaviors Among Active Duty Military Personnel, 2008

Note: Estimates are percentages among military personnel in each sociodemographic group that reported stress, depression, and generalized anxiety.

*Odds ratio is significantly different from the reference group

[a]OR=Odds ratio

OR ratios were adjusted for all other independent variables in the model

[b]95 % CI=95 % confidence interval of the odds ratio

Family status was also related to the need for further depression evaluation. The presence of a spouse appeared to be a strong protective factor against endorsing symptoms consistent with depression. Only 16.6 % (unadjusted prevalence) of personnel living with a spouse met criteria for needing further depressive evaluation, compared to 25.2 % of unmarried personnel and 25.1 % of married personnel not living with their spouse. These findings are consistent with the importance of social support as protective against symptoms of depression. In general, personnel in the lowest enlisted ranks were significantly more likely than officers to screen positive for needing further depression evaluation. Among all subgroups, personnel with the highest prevalence rates were those who reported illicit drug use in the past 30 days, those who reported getting an average of less than 4 h of nightly sleep in the past 12 months, and those who scored high on risk-taking behaviors.

When all variables were examined in the model simultaneously, the strongest risk factors for the reported depression symptoms were a positive screen for PTSD, a positive screen for GAD, and self-reported suicidal ideation in the past 12 months. Personnel with these risk factors were 3–4 times more likely to report depression symptoms than their counterparts. Personnel reporting high work or family stress or the use of avoidance coping strategies were twice as likely to report depression symptoms as those who did not report these mental health indicators. Results of this model are consistent with the literature, which indicates both a high comorbidity among mental health problems and that difficulties with coping and close interpersonal relationships are highly associated with depressive symptoms. The model also showed that personnel who slept 6 h or less on average per night over the past year had higher odds of meeting screening criteria for depression. In terms of protective factors, more frequent active coping behaviors (e.g., talking to a friend or family member) and having children living with the respondent predicted less need for depression evaluation.

5.3.3 Generalized Anxiety Disorder

Table 5.3 also shows the percentages of military personnel who met screening criteria for GAD by selected sociodemographic factors, service, and risk/protective characteristics. Overall, 14.2 % of active duty military personnel screened positive for GAD symptoms in 2008. This is consistent with other screening studies using the Patient Health Questionnaire where a range of rates was found in older samples (e.g., 4–16 %; Spitzer, Kroenke, & Williams, 1999). These rates tended to be lower than the 19.1 % prevalence rate for reporting mental health problems among service members returning from Iraq (Hoge et al., 2006). In the 2008 survey, consistent with the literature, adjusted GAD symptom screening rates decreased steadily with age. Also consistent with the literature, women, respondents with a high school education or less, and those in the lowest ranks reported the highest rates of GAD symptoms. This survey also showed that GAD symptoms varied by DoD service with personnel in the Army and Marine Corps being more likely to report GAD symptoms than personnel in the Navy or Air Force. Personnel who met criteria for GAD symptoms received less sleep, engaged in risk-taking behaviors more often, reported high levels of family stress, had been deployed, were more likely to report illness or injury in the past 12 months, had a history of physical or sexual abuse, and were more likely to engage in avoidance coping behaviors. Similar to personnel who endorsed items that suggest the need for further depressive evaluation, personnel reporting GAD symptoms also tended to screen positive for other mental health problems; GAD symptoms were 5.5 and 3.5 times more likely to be reported by personnel who screened positive for PTSD or depression, respectively. Of interest was a change from high unadjusted rates of over 20 % for illicit drug use, alcohol-related problems, and suicidal ideation in the past year, that when included in the full model, failed to be significant risk factors. This indicates that the other variables in the model accounted for any excess risk of GAD, i.e., were more important risk factors. In addition, moderate or vigorous physical exercise in the past month emerged as a significant protective factor for GAD symptoms.

5.3.4 PTSD

Table 5.4 shows the prevalence rates of PTSD, suicidal ideation in the past year, and receipt of any mental health counseling for each demographic, risk, and protective factor. As noted in Chap. 2, the conservative cutpoint of 50 on the PTSD Checklist scale used to indicate need for further PTSD evaluation was derived from samples with high prevalence rates of current PTSD and should be interpreted with caution.

In the 2008 survey, 10.7 % of DoD personnel met screening criteria for needing further PTSD evaluation in the past 30 days, compared to 6.7 % in the 2005 survey. When comparing the current (past month) rate for needing further PTSD evaluation with those in other military populations, the observed rate in the 2008 survey was 13.4 % among all Army personnel, which is slightly higher than findings from Hoge et al. (2004), which found rates of 5 % before deployment and 6.2–12.9 % after deployment. Hoge et al.'s findings reflect Army prevalence rates of PTSD several years prior to our most recent survey and are consistent with Army rates for our 2005 survey, which found an observed rate of 9.3 % for PTSD. It should be noted, however, that the population-based estimate for the Army as a whole is based on a different sociodemographic distribution than that of combat infantry personnel in the Hoge et al. (2004) study.

In our adjusted model, the strongest sociodemographic predictor of PTSD symptoms was military rank. Junior enlisted military personnel (E1–E3) across all branches of service were over 3.7 times more likely to report symptoms of PTSD than the highest-ranking officers (O4–O10). Other enlisted personnel (E4–E9) across all branches of service were also almost three times more likely than high-ranking officers to report symptoms of PTSD. Relative to African Americans, whites were at significantly less risk for PTSD. As with personnel meeting

Table 5.4 Correlates of PTSD, suicidal ideation, and mental health counseling, 2008

Independent variables	Screening positive for PTSD			Suicidal ideation			Mental health counseling		
	Unadjusted %	Adjusted %	Adjusted ORs[a] (95 % CI)[b]	Unadjusted %	Adjusted %	Adjusted ORs[a] (95 % CI)[b]	Unadjusted %	Adjusted %	Adjusted ORs[a] (95 % CI)[b]
Gender									
Male	10.5	3.4	1.00	4.5	2.4	1.00	19.2	15.8	1.00
Female	11.7	3.6	1.08 (0.87–1.35)	5.1	2.5	1.04 (0.79–1.37)	26.9	22.5	1.55* (1.39–1.73)
Age									
20 or younger	14.2	4.1	1.42 (0.85–2.38)	6.3	2.8	1.06 (0.61–1.84)	19.2	14.6	0.81 (0.54–1.20)
21–25	13.2	3.6	1.21 (0.79–1.86)	5.3	2.4	0.91 (0.63–1.31)	22.4	16.2	0.91 (0.68–1.21)
26–34	9.9	3.4	1.16 (0.79–1.69)	3.9	2.2	0.84 (0.60–1.19)	20.8	16.8	0.95 (0.76–1.18)
35 or older	6.3	3.0	1.00	3.5	2.6	1.00	17.7	17.5	1.00
Race/ethnicity									
White non-Hispanic	10.5	3.2	0.77* (0.60–0.99)	4.1	2.1	0.69* (0.48–0.99)	19.6	16.2	0.88 (0.75–1.04)
African American non-Hispanic	9.3	4.1	1.00	4.5	3.1	1.00	22.1	18.0	1.00
Hispanic	12.0	3.2	0.77 (0.54–1.08)	5.6	2.8	0.90 (0.59–1.35)	21.4	17.6	0.98 (0.81–1.18)
Other	13.0	4.6	1.13 (0.80–1.58)	7.2	3.8	1.23 (0.86–1.76)	21.3	15.9	0.87 (0.71–1.06)
Family status									
Not married	12.6	3.5	1.07 (0.88–1.30)	5.5	2.5	1.12 (0.90–1.40)	21.0	15.9	0.91 (0.80–1.04)
Married–spouse not present	12.0	3.6	1.11 (0.87–1.43)	5.2	2.9	1.27 (0.83–1.94)	22.0	16.3	0.94 (0.75–1.18)
Married–spouse present	8.6	3.3	1.00	3.7	2.3	1.00	19.5	17.2	1.00
Children living with you									
Yes	9.6	4.0	1.30* (1.05–1.60)	4.0	2.7	1.21 (0.95–1.54)	21.5	18.2	1.21* (1.07–1.38)
No	11.4	3.1	1.00	5.0	2.3	1.00	19.6	15.5	1.00
Pay grade									
E1–E3	14.6	5.0	3.76* (1.41–10.07)	6.2	2.1	1.14 (0.45–2.89)	21.9	18.7	1.97* (1.42–2.74)
E4–E6	12.4	3.7	2.80* (1.03–7.64)	4.9	2.5	1.34 (0.62–2.93)	22.6	17.5	1.82* (1.39–2.38)
E7–E9	6.4	2.7	2.02 (0.95–4.28)	3.3	2.4	1.28 (0.61–2.68)	18.1	15.9	1.62* (1.24–2.10)

W1–W5	2.9	0.5	0.38 (0.03–4.92)	3.4	3.7	1.97 (0.75–5.22)	13.7	11.6	1.12 (0.73–1.72)
O1–O3	4.7	3.5	2.58 (0.92–7.22)	2.9	2.8	1.48 (0.62–3.54)	14.0	15.1	1.52* (1.15–2.02)
O4–O10	2.6	1.4	1.00	2.2	1.9	1.00	12.0	10.5	1.00

Service

Army	13.4	3.3	1.00 (0.81–1.23)	4.9	2.3	0.98 (0.70–1.39)	24.5	17.9	1.09 (0.88–1.35)
Navy	9.2	3.3	1.01 (0.82–1.25)	5.1	2.8	1.18 (0.88–1.57)	17.7	15.0	0.88 (0.73–1.07)
Marine Corps	15.0	4.1	1.24 (0.97–1.58)	5.5	2.1	0.89 (0.68–1.16)	20.3	15.4	0.91 (0.74–1.12)
Air Force	5.6	3.3	1.00	3.1	2.4	1.00	16.2	16.7	1.00

Deployment and combat exposure

Not deployed	9.6	2.7	0.94 (0.76–1.16)	5.0	2.8	1.10 (0.76–1.60)	19.0	16.9	1.28* (1.08–1.53)
Deployed–none	6.5	2.9	1.00	4.1	2.6	1.00	14.2	13.7	1.00
Deployed–moderate	6.4	2.5	0.85 (0.66–1.10)	3.3	2.1	0.80 (0.64–1.01)	18.4	16.3	1.23* (1.07–1.42)
Deployed–high	19.6	6.9	2.50* (1.92–3.25)	5.6	2.3	0.90 (0.63–1.29)	28.6	19.5	1.53* (1.29–1.82)

Average hours of nightly sleep

7+ h	4.5	2.9	1.00	2.9	2.3	1.00	14.3	15.5	1.00
5–6 h	8.6	3.3	1.12 (0.90–1.40)	4.2	2.6	1.14 (0.90–1.46)	18.9	16.5	1.07 (0.92–1.25)
4 h or less	28.1	4.9	1.69* (1.30–2.20)	8.5	2.2	0.97 (0.70–1.36)	33.9	18.7	1.25* (1.04–1.51)

History of physical/sexual abuse

Yes	17.5	4.6	1.72* (1.42–2.09)	6.3	2.4	0.99 (0.81–1.20)	27.4	19.1	1.36* (1.17–1.57)
No	5.8	2.7	1.00	3.5	2.4	1.00	15.1	14.8	1.00

Risk-taking/impulsivity

High	27.7	3.7	1.11 (0.83–1.49)	10.8	3.1	1.33* (1.04–1.70)	33.1	18.4	1.15 (0.97–1.37)
Medium/low	9.0	3.4	1.00	4.0	2.4	1.00	19.1	16.4	1.00

Spirituality

High	8.8	4.0	1.00	4.2	2.8	1.00	20.4	18.8	1.00
Medium	10.9	3.5	0.88 (0.68–1.13)	4.3	2.3	0.83 (0.62–1.12)	20.5	16.5	0.85 (0.72–1.01)
Low	11.6	2.9	0.72* (0.55–0.93)	5.3	2.4	0.85 (0.61–1.18)	19.2	15.3	0.78* (0.61–1.00)

(continued)

Table 5.4 (continued)

Independent variables	Screening positive for PTSD			Suicidal ideation			Mental health counseling		
	Unadjusted %	Adjusted %	Adjusted ORs[a] (95 % CI)[b]	Unadjusted %	Adjusted %	Adjusted ORs[a] (95 % CI)[b]	Unadjusted %	Adjusted %	Adjusted ORs[a] (95 % CI)[b]
Moderate/vigorous physical exercise in past month									
Yes	10.6	3.5	1.14 (0.89–1.45)	4.5	2.4	1.01 (0.80–1.26)	19.6	16.1	0.80* (0.67–0.94)
No	11.1	3.1	1.00	5.4	2.4	1.00	23.8	19.4	1.00
Illness in past 12 months									
Yes	21.2	4.6	1.43* (1.12–1.83)	7.2	2.4	0.98 (0.78–1.23)	34.6	20.1	1.31* (1.15–1.50)
No	9.0	3.2	1.00	4.2	2.4	1.00	18.0	16.1	1.00
Injury in past 12 months									
Yes	14.4	3.4	1.00 (0.84–1.19)	5.5	2.5	1.04 (0.85–1.26)	26.4	19.2	1.43* (1.29–1.59)
No	7.1	3.4	1.00	3.8	2.4	1.00	14.4	14.2	1.00
Illicit drug use in past month									
Yes	23.4	4.7	1.46* (1.16–1.82)	8.3	2.4	0.98 (0.75–1.27)	34.5	19.6	1.26* (1.11–1.44)
No	9.0	3.3	1.00	4.1	2.4	1.00	18.4	16.2	1.00
Risk for alcohol-related problems									
High risk (AUDIT 8+)	20.0	4.1	1.34* (1.09–1.64)	7.4	2.3	0.93 (0.68–1.27)	27.4	17.6	1.12 (1.00–1.26)
Low risk (AUDIT <8)	6.9	3.1	1.00	3.5	2.5	1.00	17.8	16.1	1.00
Screened positive for depression									
Yes	37.4	10.2	4.47* (3.62–5.52)	13.5	6.7	3.90* (2.99–5.07)	42.9	26.1	2.09* (1.83–2.39)
No	3.4	2.5	1.00	2.2	1.8	1.00	14.0	14.5	1.00
Screened positive for generalized anxiety in past month									
Yes	47.7	13.9	5.90* (5.02–6.94)	13.2	2.6	1.08 (0.84–1.40)	43.9	18.3	1.15 (0.93–1.42)
No	4.6	2.7	1.00	3.2	2.4	1.00	16.3	16.3	1.00
Screened positive for PTSD in past month									
Yes	–	–	–	17.7	4.3	1.94* (1.58–2.38)	55.9	27.1	2.02* (1.69–2.43)
No	–	–	–	3.1	2.3	1.00	15.9	15.5	1.00

High work or family stress in past 12 months									
Yes	21.7	4.7	1.71* (1.47–1.99)	8.0	3.0	1.42* (1.06–1.91)	31.5	20.4	1.50* (1.36–1.64)
No	4.5	2.8	1.00	2.6	2.1	1.00	13.9	14.6	1.00
Suicidal ideation in past 12 months									
Yes	40.9	6.3	1.97* (1.62–2.40)	–	–	–	47.3	27.0	1.92* (1.44–2.56)
No	9.2	3.3	1.00	–	–	–	18.9	16.1	1.00
Active coping	–	–	0.80* (0.69–0.92)	–	–	0.61* (0.50–0.75)	–	–	1.02 (0.90–1.16)
Avoidance coping	–	–	1.91* (1.59–2.31)	–	–	2.32* (1.83–2.96)	–	–	1.17* (1.02–1.33)
Total	*10.7*	*10.7*	–	*4.6*	*4.6*	–	*20.3*	*20.3*	–
R^2	–	–	*0.26*	–	–	*0.07*	–	–	*0.14*

Source: DoD Survey of Health Related Behaviors Among Active Duty Military Personnel, 2008

Note: Estimates are percentages among military personnel in each sociodemographic group.

*Odds ratio is significantly different from the reference group

[a]OR = Odds ratios were adjusted for all other independent variables in the model

[b]95 % CI = 95 % confidence interval of the odds ratio

screening criteria for depression and anxiety symptoms, the subgroups with the highest prevalence rates for PTSD symptoms were personnel with additional negative mental health indicators. Personnel who screened positive for PTSD symptoms were almost six times more likely to report symptoms of GAD and were over four times more likely to report symptoms of depression. Suicidal ideation and high work or family stress were also significant risk factors. Other significant predictors of PTSD symptoms after controlling for all other variables in the model were having a history of physical or sexual abuse, illicit drug use and alcohol problems, illness, a high level of combat exposure, and an average of 4 h or less of nightly sleep in the past 12 months.

Consistent with several studies that found positive associations between avoidance coping and PTSD (e.g., Dirkzwager, Bramsen, & van der Ploeg, 2003; Fairbank, Hansen, & Fitterling, 1991; Solomon, Mikulincer, & Avitzur, 1988), avoidance coping was a moderate predictor of PTSD in the 2008 HRB survey. This expected finding is consistent with the fact that avoidance coping symptoms must be present to warrant a clinical diagnosis of PTSD. It is also not surprising that avoidance coping in general moderately predicts the presence of PTSD symptoms because other specific avoidance coping strategies, such as reported illicit drug use in the past 30 days, were also moderate predictors of PTSD symptoms. In addition, the use of active coping mechanisms was a protective factor and, somewhat unexpectedly, so was a low level of spirituality.

5.3.5 Suicidal Ideation

Greater attention has been paid to suicide in the military since an update of the Army's Mental Health Advisory Team report found that suicide rates for soldiers deployed to Iraq have remained above normal levels since 2003 (Office of the Surgeon, 2008). Rates across the Army and veteran populations are now higher than the national average and are comorbid with other mental health problems (U.S. Army, 2012). Findings from the 2008 survey showed that 4.6 % of DoD personnel reported seriously considering suicide and 2.2 % reported a suicide attempt in the past year. The 2005 rate for suicide contemplation (4.9 %) was similar to that for 2008, but the 2005 rate for suicide attempts (0.8 %) was significantly lower than in the 2008 survey. Prior to joining the military, almost 4 % of personnel had seriously considered suicide and about 3 % had attempted suicide.

Table 5.4 shows the estimated prevalence rates for past year suicidal ideation by sociodemographic characteristics and risk and protective factors. The highest unadjusted prevalence rates were seen among personnel who met screening criteria for PTSD, had depression symptoms, and had GAD symptoms, followed by those who reported engaging in risk-taking behaviors. After adjusting for all the variables in the model, depression, avoidance coping, and PTSD were the strongest predictors of suicidal ideation. Those screening positive for depression were nearly four times more likely to have suicidal thoughts than those not meeting criteria. Personnel who engaged in avoidance coping, which included thinking of suicide when stressed, were 2.32 times as likely as those with lower scores to have seriously considered suicide in the past year, and those screening positive for PTSD were nearly twice as likely to have suicidal thoughts as their counterparts who did not meet criteria. High work or family stress and high risk-taking were also significant risk factors. Active coping was found to be a protective factor against suicidal ideation; personnel who engaged in active coping strategies were approximately half as likely to consider suicide as those who did not. It should also be noted that despite the large number of potential risk and protective factors examined in the model, only 7 % of the variance was accounted for, indicating that other factors not measured are impacting the risk of suicidal ideation in the military.

5.3.6   Mental Health Counseling

In addition to describing the epidemiology of psychological problems among DoD personnel, the 2008 HRB survey examined rates of mental health treatment utilization. Specifically, beyond tracking changes in the receipt of mental health counseling as described above, this survey sought to capture information about treatment issues, such as which personnel perceived the need for psychological treatment, which personnel received mental health counseling, why personnel sought psychological treatment, and how personnel perceived that seeking treatment could potentially affect their military career.

Respondents in the 2008 HRB survey were asked whether they felt they needed mental health counseling within the past 12 months, whether they had received such care, and reasons for seeking it. Overall, 19.8 % of personnel perceived a need for mental health counseling in the past year. A reported 20 % of personnel received counseling or therapy for mental health or substance abuse from a professional health care provider, chaplain or other pastoral counselor, or self-help group. Personnel reported receiving counseling most frequently from a military mental health professional (10.2 %), a general physician at a military facility (7.3 %), or a military chaplain (6.1 %). Respondents perceived the need for mental health counseling significantly more in the 2008 survey than in the 2005 survey (19.8 % vs. 17.8 %). Respondents sought help most frequently for depression (7.8 %), anxiety (5.9 %), and family problems (7.5 %).

As shown in Table 5.4, the strongest predictors for seeking mental health counseling were meeting screening criteria for PTSD or depression and reporting suicidal ideation. Those positive for each of these variables were approximately twice as likely to obtain mental health counseling as their counterparts. Other significant predictors of seeking mental health counseling were illicit drug use in the past 30 days, having an illness or injury in the past 12 months, getting 4 or fewer hours of nightly sleep, scoring high on a measure of risk-taking behaviors, having a history of physical or sexual abuse, and reporting high work or family stress. Among sociodemographic groups, women were most likely to have sought help. Additional factors associated with receipt of counseling included being enlisted and having children living with the service member. Of note, having moderate to high combat exposure or not being deployed at all were also significant predictors of seeking mental health counseling, the latter most likely indicating that the personnel were screened out of pre-deployment qualification. A low score on spirituality was predictive of non-receipt of mental health services.

Personnel were also questioned about whether they thought that mental health counseling would have a detrimental impact on their military career. More personnel perceived that counseling "definitely or probably would not" damage a military career (63.9 %) compared to those who perceived that it "definitely or probably would" damage a military career (36.1 %). This pattern was fairly consistent across the four services. Those personnel who perceived that receiving mental health counseling "definitely or probably would not" damage their career increased significantly from 2005 to 2008 (55.8 % vs. 63.9 %) at least partially reflecting changing perceptions about the stigma associated with receiving mental health treatment in the military. However, even with improving perceptions that receiving mental health care would not damage one's military career, still over one third of personnel did not hold that view.

To determine whether the perception of negative repercussions is deterring some personnel from receiving mental health counseling, the opinions of those who indicated a need for this type of treatment were examined. If personnel who needed treatment and received it perceived more positive career outcomes, this would indicate that these fears are largely unwarranted. If, however, those who had received mental health treatment perceived a greater threat to their career than those who had not received treatment, this would indicate that they may have experienced negative career consequences as a result of their counseling.

Figure 5.4 includes data only for those who perceived a need for mental health services, revealed a need for further anxiety or depression evaluation, or reported suicidal ideation in the past 12 months. Thus, this is a small subset of active duty personnel. Within each group, respondents were divided into those who had received mental health counseling in the past 12 months and those who had not. As shown, among those who felt they needed counseling, those who had not received mental health services (53.2 %) were more likely than those who had received them (47.3 %) to respond that such services "definitely or probably would" damage a person's military career. In contrast, personnel who had received mental health counseling (52.7 %) were more likely than those who had not received such services (46.8 %) to respond that such services "probably or definitely would not" damage a person's career. Among personnel who met criteria for depression, GAD symptoms, or suicidal ideation, those who had not received mental health services were just as likely as or less likely than those who had received them to perceive damage to their career as a result of seeking services. Thus, personnel who received services were generally more likely to believe that having done so would not have a negative impact on their career compared to those who did not receive such services. However, among personnel needing further mental health evaluation who did receive services, less than half perceived that this would not damage their career (e.g., 44.0 % GAD symptoms, 46.1 % depression evaluation, 36.3 % suicidal ideation). In other words, there was still strong concern even among those who received treatment.

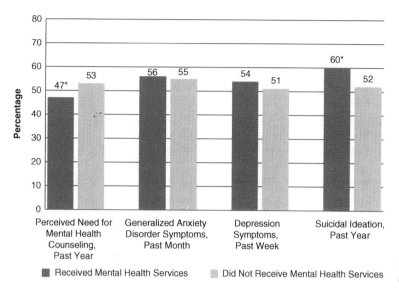

Fig. 5.4 Perceived damage to military career for seeking mental health services among DoD personnel, by selected mental health measures, 2008
*Estimate is significantly different from the "Did Not Receive Mental Health Services" estimate at the 0.05 level

5.4 Summary and Discussion

This chapter examined trends, prevalence, and risk and protective factors for a variety of mental health issues and problems among military personnel. These include stress, coping mechanisms, symptoms of anxiety and depression, PTSD, suicidal ideation, and perceptions and receipt of mental health counseling.

5.4.1 Levels and Sources of Stress

Overall, work and family stress levels in the active duty military have declined between 1988 and 2008. A higher percentage of military personnel rated their jobs as more stressful than their personal lives. The reasons for the recent decreases in work and family stress compared with previous surveys are unclear and may be numerous. There are several explanations that seem particularly plausible. The first may be the success of DoD's attempts to mitigate stress on active duty personnel through stress-reduction interventions or resilience training (see Meredith et al., 2011, for a review of military resilience programs). A second is that service members may have adapted to the stressors in their environment such that events that were stressful in earlier years have become more routine (see also Bray et al., 2010). It is also possible that recruits during wartime are different than those prior to the recent conflicts and self-select into the military with the understanding that they will be sent into combat as opposed to recruits during peacetime who may not have expected to be involved in combat and consequently perceived greater work-related stress. Additional research is needed to unravel the underlying mechanism(s).

The most frequently cited stressful events were family separations, deployments, and increases in work load. That these stressors rank high is understandable in the context of the intense military involvements in the Iraq and Afghanistan conflicts that have been ongoing for over a decade. Our findings that depression and anxiety were the strongest predictors of work or family stress suggest that efforts to address these mental health problems may also have a positive effect on reducing stress. Without question, a military wartime environment results in enhanced stress for service members and their families. They point to the need for effective stress-reduction training, a better understanding of the factors that lead service members and families to engage in positive coping behaviors, and the availability of strong support groups and programs.

5.4.2   Coping with Stress

Recent increases in reported stress related to numerous life events raise the question of how military personnel are coping with stress and whether coping strategies can be improved to help reduce the experience of stress. Coping has been defined in terms of the strategies and processes that individuals use to modify adverse aspects of their environment as well as to minimize internal distress induced by environmental demands (Lazarus, 1966; Moos & Billings, 1982). An important dimension of coping is the distinction between active coping, such as problem-focused coping strategies (efforts to recognize, modify, or eliminate the impact of a stressor) and emotion-focused coping strategies (efforts to regulate negative emotions that occur in reaction to a stressor event), and avoidance coping strategies (efforts to avoid dealing with the stressor). Although the utility of any approach depends on the demands of the situation and the skill and flexibility of individuals in using various coping strategies, preference for an avoidance strategy has been linked with a greater risk of mental health problems in military personnel, especially when individuals are faced with a radically changing environment (Johnsen, Laberg, & Eid, 1998). Similarly, higher use of active coping strategies has been found to be related to lower levels of psychological symptoms among Gulf War Army personnel (Sharkansky et al., 2000).

The 2008 HRB survey showed that military personnel tended to use more constructive active coping strategies than avoidance-oriented strategies. The most commonly used strategies for coping with stress were thinking of a plan to solve the problem, seeking social support by talking to a friend or family member, and engaging in physical activity and/or a hobby. These encouraging findings are tempered somewhat by the findings that approximately one-third of military personnel report using alcohol as a coping strategy and more than one-quarter of military personnel commonly use tobacco to cope with stress, daily pressures, and feelings of depression.

5.4.3 Mental Health Indicators

A major strength of HRB data has been the rare opportunity to examine the overlap in prevalence among various mental health problems. Overall, our findings point to a striking comorbidity among the mental health indicators that were studied. Among the large number of potential risk factors examined as predictors of mental health indicators, two factors predicted all mental health outcomes: use of avoidance coping and high levels of work or family stress. Two other factors—an average of 4 or fewer hours of nightly sleep and a history of physical or sexual abuse—were also significant predictors of all mental health outcomes except for suicidal ideation.

In addition to identifying risk factors for negative psychological outcomes, our analyses identified protective factors that may buffer against the development of common mental health problems experienced by military personnel. Our findings indicated that use of active coping strategies is the primary protective factor against negative mental health outcomes; in particular, active coping was associated with all mental health outcomes except high stress and anxiety. Military personnel who report using avoidance coping strategies are most likely to suffer from negative mental health consequences, whereas those who implement active coping strategies appear least likely to develop mental health problems. The somewhat unexpected finding that a low score on spirituality was protective against PTSD and predictive of non-receipt of mental health services suggests that those with low spirituality may be more immune to the moral dilemmas and conflicts often presented by warfare and are less apt to seek help. Thus, our analyses indicate that further study into the particular mechanisms of action behind the protective mental health effects of active coping and spirituality is warranted. Specific findings related to the outcomes are summarized below.

Prevalence estimates from the HRB survey indicate that symptoms of depression occur more frequently in active duty military personnel than in the civilian population. In the civilian population, the *lifetime* prevalence of experiencing a depressive episode is approximately 17 % in men and 21 % in women (Kessler et al., 1994). Prevalence rates for current (past week) depressive symptoms for military men and women were 20.4 and 25.7 %, respectively. Because lifetime prevalence rates are expected to be higher than rates for the past 7 days, they strongly suggest that depression in military men and women has become more common in the military than civilian populations at least during wartime. Gender differences in depression were similar to those reported in the civilian population (Burt, 2002; Kessler et al., 1994) with a higher percentage of military women scoring above the thresholds on the depression screeners.

Estimates from a community sample indicate that the 1-year prevalence rate for GAD was approximately 3 % (American Psychiatric Association, 1994). Reports of GAD symptoms are markedly higher in military personnel (14.2 %) as measured by the screeners used in the 2008 survey. It should be reiterated that these screeners do not provide a diagnosis of the disorder, but rather indicate the need for further evaluation and may reflect differences from community sample estimates based on different measures, different screening criteria, and different time periods between surveys. Military women also reported more symptoms of GAD compared to their male counterparts, which is consistent with estimates in national psychiatric epidemiological studies (Kessler et al., 1994).

For both men and women, a similar profile of risk factors was observed for those meeting screening criteria for depression and anxiety, although some noteworthy differences were evident. Inadequate sleep (less than 4 h per night) was a significant risk factor for both depressive and anxiety symptoms, as was a history of physical or sexual abuse, having an injury in the past 12 months, reporting high work or family stress, and using avoidance coping behaviors. On the other hand, although not having a spouse present and being a member of the Navy were risk factors for depressive symptoms but not anxiety symptoms, combat exposure, having an illness in the past 12 months, being white, and scoring high on risk-taking increased the risk of anxiety symptoms but not depressive symptoms. Further, whereas younger age, living with children, and using active coping mechanisms were protective for depression symptoms, only moderate or vigorous physical exercise in the past month was a significant protective factor for anxiety symptoms.

The finding that a considerable proportion of military personnel met screening criteria for depression and anxiety symptoms is not surprising. Depressive disorders and anxiety disorders such as GAD are among the most common mental health problems in the general population and among military personnel returning from Iraq (Hoge et al., 2004). Depressive and anxiety disorders are also serious negative mental health outcomes that, if left untreated, pose serious health consequences to veterans, that negatively affect mission readiness and are related to recent attrition (Hoge et al., 2006). However, it is important to note that differences in risk factors may be used to help target screening efforts for at-risk personnel. Also, these data suggest that there are specific protective factors, such as exercise, that may be used to improve intervention efforts.

In addition to the serious health risk posed by depression and anxiety disorders, PTSD is an anxiety disorder that presents another negative mental health consequence for which military personnel are particularly vulnerable. Community-based samples place the lifetime prevalence of PTSD at a lower rate than at-risk samples, which include groups such as combat veterans and other victims of trauma. Community-based samples generally range from 1 to 14 %, whereas at-risk samples vary greatly between 3 and 58 % according to the Diagnostic Statistical Manual (DSM-IV) (American Psychiatric Association, 1994). The HRB data showed a marked but not surprising increasing in the prevalence of PTSD between 2005 and 2008. Although the HRB survey is the first to assess PTSD within the total active force, the increase in estimated rates is consistent with the large amount of literature on returning OIF/OEF Soldiers and Marines (e.g., Hoge et al., 2006; Tanielian et al., 2008) and may be indicative of both combat exposure and/or an increase in recruits with prior traumatic exposures. We found that several risk factors are unique to PTSD in the military as a whole. Junior enlisted rank, illicit drug use in the past 30 days, and a history of physical or sexual abuse prior to joining the military place active duty personnel at higher risk for experiencing PTSD symptoms. In addition to other reasons, it is possible that military personnel in the lowest enlisted ranks (E1–E3) are at the highest risk for developing PTSD symptoms because these personnel may be most likely to be exposed to traumatic experiences during deployment (e.g., combat situations). Illicit drug use is also a significant risk factor for PTSD; however, it is unclear whether drug use actually makes personnel more vulnerable to experiencing PTSD symptoms after witnessing a trauma or whether personnel may "self-medicate" in response to exposure to a traumatic event, which in turn impedes the recovery process and leads to increased PTSD symptoms. This distinction warrants additional investigation. Finally, military personnel with a history of physical or sexual abuse are at heightened risk for reporting PTSD symptoms. This finding is consistent with literature that suggests prior or repeated traumatic exposures render individuals at greater risk for PTSD after subsequent traumatic exposures.

The finding that slightly more DoD personnel reported seriously considering suicide during active duty (4.6 %) than prior to joining the military suggests that some personnel come into the service potentially vulnerable to suicidal ideation and that active duty experience may increase their risk. Despite these concerns, the findings that avoidance coping was the strongest predictor of suicidal ideation and that personnel who engaged in more active coping were approximately half as likely as those who engaged in more avoidance coping to have seriously considered suicide suggests that interventions designed to improve coping skills may help reduce the number of at-risk personnel.

Our findings about the substantial comorbidities among mental health problems raise many questions about the types and intensity of interventions that are needed to address these overlapping and complex problems and point to the need for additional research in this arena. As an initial step, we are currently engaged in further investigation to characterize the specific degree of overlap among indicators and develop separate profiles for each comorbid pattern.

5.4.4 Mental Health Services Utilization

Approximately 20 % of personnel perceived a need for mental health counseling in the 12 months prior to the survey, and approximately the same percentage of personnel received care. This is in contrast to the findings of the 2002 HRB survey (Bray et al., 2003) in which a similar percentage perceived a need for treatment (18.7 %) but only 12.5 % received care. This suggests that the gap between the perceived need for treatment and receipt of treatment may be shrinking. Nonetheless, a large portion of personnel still believed that receiving counseling may be detrimental to one's career, which likely leads to a continued reluctance to receive mental health counseling. To facilitate appropriate help-seeking behavior and targeted interventions, further research is needed to characterize those who are screening positive for mental health problems but who do not perceive a need for treatment or seek treatment.

In light of these findings, it is possible that the military's efforts in recent years to reduce the stigma associated with receiving mental health counseling have at least partially succeeded. One step in this process has been to increase awareness of the importance of mental fitness. Mental health has been recognized as an essential aspect of military readiness; recent directives have specified routine medical surveillance (including mental health) for active duty service members (DoD, 1997b) to monitor the health of this population and intervene when necessary. Under this policy, all service members must be mentally fit to carry out their missions, and their mental health must be maintained, assessed, and protected. In addition, the rights of service members referred for mental health evaluation are protected (DoD, 1997a; Litts & Roadman, 1997). Recent thinking also recommends a new total force fitness paradigm that broadens fitness across eight different domains that specifically include mental health fitness (Jonas et al., 2010). Limited empirical evidence also suggests that mental health evaluation will not necessarily have a negative impact on an individual's military career. For example, in a small survey of 138 commanding and executive officers in the Navy and Marine Corps, the majority of officers reported a neutral view of service members who received mental health counseling (Porter & Johnson, 1994). Despite these potentially encouraging steps, more efforts are needed to combat the widely held concern that seeking help for psychological problems will have negative career consequences.

5.5   Recap

This chapter has described results from stress and mental health screening measures used for active duty DoD personnel. These measures were incorporated into recent iterations of the HRB survey in 2005 and 2008 in response to the growing concern over stress and mental health conditions that troops face during and after their return from deployment in Iraq and Afghanistan. Our goal has been to move current research in this important field forward by providing the most current prevalence estimates using population-based data for high levels of family and work stress as well as mental health conditions such as depression, GAD, PTSD, and suicidality. These data help identify the serious negative mental health consequences that affect military personnel most frequently, the risk and protective factors associated with such consequences, and the comorbid nature of these mental health problems. Identification of changing prevalence estimates and groups at risk for certain mental health conditions provides an important step toward the development, improvement, and implementation of appropriate and effective treatments.

References

Adler, A. B., Bliese, P. D., & Castro, C. A. (Eds.). (2011). *Deployment psychology*. Washington, DC: American Psychological Association.
American Psychiatric Association. (1994). *Diagnostic and statistical manual of mental disorders* (4th ed.). Washington, DC: Author.

American Psychological Association, Presidential Task Force on Military Deployment Services for Youth, Families and Service Members. (2007). *The psychological needs of U.S. military service members and their families: A preliminary report.* http://www.ptsd.ne.gov/publications/military-deployment-task-force-report.pdf

Black, D. W., Carney, C. P., Forman-Hoffman, V. L., Letuchy, E., Pelosdo, P., Woolson, R. F., et al. (2004). Depression in veterans of the first Gulf War and comparable military controls. *Annals of Clinical Psychiatry, 16*, 53–61.

Bolton, E. E. (2001). Reports of prior exposure to potentially traumatic events and PTSD in troops posed for deployment. *Journal of Traumatic Stress, 14*(1), 249–256.

Booth-Kewley, S., & Larson, G. E. (2005). Predictors of psychiatric hospitalization in the Navy. *Military Medicine, 170*(1), 87–93.

Bray, R. M., Hourani, L. L., Rae, K. L., Dever, J. A., Brown, J. M., Vincus, A. A., et al. (2003). *2002 Department of Defense survey of health related behaviors among military personnel: Final report* (prepared for the Assistant Secretary of Defense [Health Affairs], U.S. Department of Defense, Cooperative Agreement No. DAMD17-00-2-0057/RTI/7841/ 006-FR). Research Triangle Park, NC: Research Triangle Institute.

Bray, R. M., Hourani, L. L., Rae Olmsted, K. L., Witt, M., Brown, J. M., Pemberton, M. R., et al. (2006). *2005 Department of Defense survey of health related behaviors among active duty military personnel* (RTI/7841/106-FR). Research Triangle Park, NC: Research Triangle Institute.

Bray, R. M., Kroutil, L. A., Luckey, J. W., Wheeless, S. C., Iannacchione, V. G., Anderson, D. W., et al. (1992). *1992 worldwide survey of substance abuse and health behaviors among military personnel.* Research Triangle Park, NC: Research Triangle Institute.

Bray, R. M., Kroutil, L. A., Wheeless, S. C., Marsden, M. E., Bailey, S. L., Fairbank, J. A., et al. (1995). *1995 Department of Defense Survey of health related behaviors among military personnel* (DoD Contract No. DASO1-94-C-0140). Research Triangle Park, NC: Research Triangle Institute.

Bray, R. M., Marsden, M. E., Guess, L. L., Wheeless, S. C., Iannacchione, V. G., & Keesling, S. R. (1988). *1988 worldwide survey of substance abuse and health behaviors among military personnel.* Research Triangle Park, NC: Research Triangle Institute.

Bray, R. M., Pemberton, M. R., Hourani, L. L., Witt, M., Rae Olmsted, K. L., Brown, J. M., et al. (2009). *2008 Department of Defense survey of health related behaviors among active duty military personnel.* Report prepared for TRICARE Management Activity, Office of the Assistant Secretary of Defense (Health Affairs) and U.S. Coast Guard. Research Triangle Park, NC: Research Triangle Institute.

Bray, R. M., Pemberton, M. R., Lane, M. E., Hourani, L. L., Mattiko, M. J., & Babeu, L. A. (2010). Substance use and mental health trends among U.S. military active duty personnel: Key findings from the 2008 DoD Health Behavior Survey. *Military Medicine, 175*, 390–399.

Bray, R. M., Sanchez, R. P., Ornstein, M. L., Lentine, D., Vincus, A. A., Baird, T. U., et al. (1999). *1998 Department of Defense survey of health related behaviors among military personnel: Final report* (prepared for the Assistant Secretary of Defense [Health Affairs], U.S. Department of Defense, Cooperative Agreement No. DAMD17-96-2-6021, RTI/7034/006-FR). Research Triangle Park, NC: Research Triangle Institute.

Britt, T. W., Greene-Shortridge, T. M., Brink, S., Nguyen, Q. B., Rath, J., Cox, A. L., et al. (2008). Perceived stigma and barriers to care for psychological treatment: Implications for reactions to stressors in different contexts. *Journal of Social and Clinical Psychology, 27*(4), 317–335.

Britt, T. W., Greene-Shortridge, T. M., & Castro, C. A. (2007). The stigma of mental health problems in the military. *Military Medicine, 172*, 157–161.

Burnam, A., Meredith, L. S., Tanielian, T., & Jaycox, L. H. (2009). Mental health care for Iraq and Afghanistan War veterans. *Health Affairs, 28*(3), 771–782.

Burrell, L. M., Durand, D. B., & Castro, C. A. (2006). The impact of military lifestyle demands on well-being, army, and family outcomes. *Armed Forces & Society, 33*, 43–58.

Burt, V. K. (2002). Women and depression: Special considerations in assessment and management. In F. Lewis-Hall, T. S. Williams, J. A. Panetta, & J. M. Herrera (Eds.), *Psychiatric illness in women* (pp. 113–116). Washington, DC: American Psychological Publishing.

Carbone, E. G., & Cigrang, J. A. (2001). Job satisfaction, occupational stress, and personality characteristics of Air Force military training instructors. *Military Medicine, 166*(9), 800–802.

Department of Defense. (1997a). *Directive No. 6490.1. Mental health evaluations of members of the armed forces* (for full on-line text, see http://web7.whs.osd.mil/text/d64902p.txt). Washington, DC: Author.

Department of Defense. (1997b). *Directive No. 6490.2: Joint medical surveillance* (for full on-line text, see http://web7.whs.osd.mil/text/d64902.txt). Washington, DC: Author.

Department of Defense Task Force on Mental Health. (2007). *An achievable vision: Report of the Department of Defense Task Force on Mental Health.* Falls Church, VA: Defense Health Board.

Desai, M. M., Rosenheck, R. A., & Desai, R. A. (2008). Time trends and predictors of suicide among mental health outpatients in the Department of Veterans Affairs. *Journal of Behavioral Health Services & Research, 35*(1), 115–124.

Dirkzwager, A., Bramsen, I., & van der Ploeg, H. (2003). Social support, coping, life events, and posttraumatic stress symptoms among former peacekeepers: A prospective study. *Personality and Individual Differences, 8*, 1545–1559.

Dohrenwend, B. P., Turner, J. B., Turse, N. A., Adams, B. G., Koenen, K. C., & Marshall, R. (2006). The psychological risks of Vietnam for U.S. veterans: A revisit with new data and methods. *Science, 313*, 979–982.

Dolan, C. A., & Adler, A. B. (2006). Military hardiness as a buffer of psychological health on return from deployment. *Military Medicine, 171*, 93–98.

Dolan, C. A., Adler, A. B., Thomas, J. L., & Castro, C. A. (2005). Operations tempo and soldier health: The moderating effect of wellness behavior. *Military Psychology, 17*(3), 157–174.

Dolan, C. A., & Ender, M. G. (2008). The coping paradox: Work, stress, and coping in the U.S. army. *Military Psychology, 20*(3), 151–169.

Elsass, W. P. (2001). Susceptibility to maladaptive responses to stress in basic military training based on variants of temperament and character. *Military Medicine, 166*, 884–888.

Fairbank, J. A., Hansen, D. J., & Fitterling, J. M. (1991). Patterns of appraisal and coping across different stressor conditions among former prisoners of war with and without posttraumatic stress disorder. *Journal of Consulting and Clinical Psychology, 50*, 274–281.

Foa, E. B., Steketee, G., & Olasov Rothbaum, B. (1989). Behavioral/cognitive conceptualizations of post-traumatic stress disorder. *Behavior Therapy, 20*, 155–176.

Folkman, S., & Lazarus, R. S. (1980). An analysis of coping in a middle-aged community sample. *Journal of Health and Social Behavior, 21*, 219–239.

Folkman, S., & Lazarus, R. S. (1985). If it changes, it must be a process: Study of emotion and coping during three stages of a college examination. *Journal of Personality and Social Psychology, 48*, 150–170.

Grieger, T. A., Cozza, S. J., Ursano, R. J., Hoge, C., Martinez, P. E., Engel, C. C., et al. (2006). Posttraumatic stress disorder and depression in battle-injured soldiers. *American Journal of Psychiatry, 163*, 1777–1783.

Gunderson, E. K., & Hourani, L. L. (2001a). The epidemiology of mental disorders in the U.S. Navy: The neuroses. *Military Medicine, 166*(7), 612–620.

Gunderson, E. K., & Hourani, L. L. (2001b). The epidemiology of mental disorders in the U.S. Navy: The psychoses. *Military Psychology, 13*(2), 99–116.

Gunderson, E. K., & Hourani, L. L. (2003). The epidemiology of personality disorders in the U.S. Navy. *Military Medicine, 168*(7), 575–582.

Henning, K. R., & Frueh, B. C. (1997). Combat guilt and its relationship PTSD symptoms. *Journal of Clinical Psychology, 53*(8), 801–808.

Hoge, C. W., Auchterlonie, J. L., & Milliken, C. S. (2006). Mental health problems, use of mental health services, and attrition from military service after returning from deployment to Iraq or Afghanistan. *Journal of the American Medical Association, 295*, 1023–1032.

Hoge, C. W., Castro, C. A., Messer, S. C., McGurk, D., Cotting, D. I., & Koffman, R. L. (2004). Combat duty in Iraq and Afghanistan, mental health problems, and barriers to care. *New England Journal of Medicine, 351*, 13–22.

Hoge, C. W., Lesikar, S. E., Guevera, R., Lange, J., Brundage, J. F., Engel, C. C., et al. (2002). Mental disorders among US military personnel in the 1990s: Association with high levels of health care utilization and early military attrition. *American Journal of Psychiatry, 159*, 1576–1583.

Hoge, C. W., Toboni, H. E., Messer, S. C., Bell, N., Amoroso, P., & Orman, D. T. (2005). The occupational burden of mental disorders in the U.S. military: Psychiatric hospitalizations, involuntary separations, and disability. *American Journal of Psychiatry, 162*, 585–591.

Hourani, L. L., Davidson, L., Clinton-Sherrod, M., Patel, N., Marshall, M., & Crosby, A. E. (2006). Suicide prevention and community-level indictors. *Evaluation and Program Planning, 29*(4), 377–385.

Hourani, L., Yuan, H., & Bray, R. (2003). Psychosocial and health correlates of types of traumatic event exposures among U.S. military personnel. *Military Medicine, 168*(9), 737–743.

Johnsen, B. H., Laberg, J. C., & Eid, J. (1998). Coping strategies and mental health problems in a military unit. *Military Medicine, 163*, 599–602.

Jonas, W. B., O'Connor, F. G., Deuster, P., Peck, J., Shake, C., & Frost, S. S. (2010). Why total force fitness? *Military Medicine, 175*(1), 6–13.

Jones, D. E., Kennedy, K. R., & Hourani, L. L. (2006). Suicide prevention in the military. In C. H. Kennedy & E. A. Zillmer (Eds.), *Military psychology: Clinical and operational applications* (pp. 130–162). New York: The Guilford Press.

Jones, E., & Wessely, S. C. (2005). *Shell shock to PTSD: Military psychiatry from 1900 to the Gulf War*. Hove, England: Psychology Press.

Kennedy, C. H., & McNeil, J. A. (2006). A history of military psychology. In C. H. Kennedy & E. A. Zillmer (Eds.), *Military psychology: Clinical and operational applications* (pp. 1–17). New York: The Guilford Press.

Kessler, R. C., McGonagle, K. A., Zhao, S., Nelson, C. B., Hughes, M., Eshleman, S., et al. (1994). Lifetime and 12-month prevalence of DSM-III-R psychiatric disorders in the United States. Results from the National Comorbidity Survey. *Archives of General Psychiatry, 51*, 8–19.

Kress, A. M., Peterson, M. R., & Hartzell, M. C. (2006). Association between obesity and depressive symptoms among U.S. Military active duty service personnel, 2002. *Journal of Psychosomatic Research, 60*(3), 263–271.

Langston, V., & Gould, M. (2007). Culture: What is its effect on stress in the military? *Military Medicine, 172*, 931–935.

Lazarus, R. S. (1966). *Psychological stress and the coping process*. New York: McGraw-Hill.

Levy, B. S., & Sidel, V. W. (2009). Health effects of combat: A life-course perspective. *Annual Review of Public Health, 30*, 123–136.

Litts, D. (Lt Col, HQ AFMOA/SGOC), & Roadman, C. H. I. (Lt General, USAF, MC, Surgeon General). (1997). *Mental health and military law* (Air Force Instruction 44-109). Washington, DC: Secretary of the Air Force.

Litz, B. T. (2007). Research on the impact of military trauma: Current status and future directions. *Military Psychology, 19*, 217–238.

MacGregor, A. J., Shaffer, R. A., Dougherty, A. L., Galarneau, M. R., Raman, R., Baker, D. G., et al. (2009). Psychological correlates of battle and nonbattle injury among Operation Iraqi Freedom veterans. *Military Medicine, 174*(3), 224–231.

Maguen, S., Suvak, M., & Litz, B. T. (2006). Predictors and prevalence of posttraumatic stress disorder among military veterans. In A. B. Adler, C. A. Castro, & T. W. Britt (Eds.), *Military life: The psychology of serving in peace and combat* (Vol. 2, pp. 141–169). Westport, CT: Praeger Security International.

Marmar, C. R. (2009). Mental health impact of Afghanistan and Iraq deployment: Meeting the challenge of a new generation of veterans. *Depression and Anxiety, 26*(6), 493–497.

Martin, L., Rosen, L. N., Durant, D. B., Knudson, K. H., & Stretch, R. H. (2000). Psychological and physical health effects of sexual assaults and nonsexual traumas among male and female United States Army soldiers. *Behavioral Medicine, 26*, 23–33.

McFarlane, A. C. (2009). The duration of deployment and sensitization to stress. *Psychiatric Annals, 39*(2), 81–88.

Meredith, L. S., Sherbourne, C. A., Gaillot, S., Hansell, L., Ritchard, H. V., Parker, A. M., et al. (2011). *Promoting psychological resilience in the U.S. Military. Rand Center for Military Health Policy Research.* Santa Monica, CA: Rand Corporation.

Moore, B. A., & Reger, G. M. (2007). Historical and contemporary perspectives of combat stress and the Army combat stress control team. In C. R. Figley & W. P. Nash (Eds.), *Combat stress injury: Theory, research, and management* (pp. 161–181). New York: Routledge.

Moos, R., & Billings, A. (1982). Conceptualizing and measuring coping resources and processes. In L. Goldberger & S. Breznitz (Eds.), *Handbook of stress: Theoretical and clinical aspects* (pp. 212–230). New York: Macmillan.

Nash, W. P. (2007a). The stressors of war. In C. F. Figley & W. P. Nash (Eds.), *Combat stress injury: Theory, research, and management* (pp. 11–31). New York: Routledge.

Nash, W. P. (2007b). Combat/operational stress adaptations and injuries. In C. F. Figley & W. P. Nash (Eds.), *Combat stress injury: Theory, research, and management* (pp. 33–63). New York: Routledge.

Office of the Surgeon Multinational Force-Iraq and Office of the Surgeon General United States Army Medical Command Mental Health Advisory Team (MHAT) IV. (2006). *Operation Iraqi Freedom 05-07 final report.* http://www.griegermd.com/MHAT_IV_Consolidated_Report.pdf

Office of the Surgeon Multinational Force-Iraq and Office of the Surgeon General United States Army Medical Command, Mental Health Advisory Team (MHAT) V. (2008). *Operation Iraqi Freedom 06-08: Iraq.* http://armymedicine.mil/Documents/Redacted1-MHATV-OIF-4-FEB-2008Report.pdf

Orasanu, J. M., & Backer, P. (1996). Stress and military performance. In J. E. Driskell & E. Salas (Eds.), *Stress and human performance* (pp. 89–125). Mahwah, NJ: Lawrence Erlbaum Associates.

Owens, G. P., Dashevsky, B., Chard, K. M., Mohamed, S., Haji, U., Heppner, P. S., et al. (2009). The relationship between childhood trauma, combat exposure, and posttraumatic stress disorder in male veterans. *Military Psychology, 21*(1), 114–125.

Pflanz, S. (2001). Occupational stress and psychiatric illness in the military: Investigation of the relationship between occupational stress and mental illness among military mental health patients. *Military Medicine, 166,* 457–462.

Pflanz, S., & Sonnek, S. (2002). Work stress in the military: Prevalence, causes, and relationship to emotional health. *Military Medicine, 167,* 877–882.

Pietrzak, R. H., Johnson, D. C., Goldstein, M. B., Malley, J. C., & Southwick, S. M. (2009). Perceived stigma and barriers to mental health care utilization among OEF-OIF veterans. *Psychiatric Services, 60*(8), 1118–1122.

Pols, H., & Oak, S. (2007). War & military mental health: The U.S. psychiatric response in the 20th century. *American Journal of Public Health, 97*(12), 2132–2142.

Porter, T. L., & Johnson, W. B. (1994). Psychiatric stigma in the military. *Military Medicine, 159,* 602–605.

Regier, D. A., Famer, M. E., Rae, D. S., Locke, B. Z., Keith, S. J., Judd, L. L., et al. (1990). Comorbidity of mental disorders with alcohol and other drug abuse: Results from the Epidemiologic Catchment Area (ECA) study. *Journal of the American Medical Association, 264,* 2511–2518.

Riddle, M. S., Sandersa, J. W., Jones, J. J., & Webb, S. C. (2008). Self-reported combat stress indicators among troops deployed to Iraq and Afghanistan: An epidemiological study. *Comprehensive Psychiatry, 49*(4), 340–345.

Ritchie, E. C., Keppler, W. C., & Rothberg, J. M. (2003). Suicidal admission in the United States Military. *Military Medicine, 168,* 177–181.

Rona, R. J., Fear, N. T., Hull, L., Greenberg, N., Earnshaw, M., Hotopf, M., et al. (2008). Mental health consequences of overstretch in the UK armed forces: First phase of a cohort study. *BMJ, 335*(7620), 603.

Rosen, L. N., Wright, K., Marlowe, D., Bartone, P., & Gifford, R. K. (1999). Gender differences in subjective distress attributable to anticipation of combat among U.S. Army soldiers deployed to the Persian Gulf during Operation Desert Storm. *Military Medicine, 164,* 753–757.

Safran, M. A., Strine, T. W., Dhingra, S. S., Berry, J. T., Manderscheid, R., & Mokdad, A. H. (2009). Psychological distress and mental health treatment among persons with and without active duty military experience, Behavioral Risk Factor Surveillance System, United States, 2007. *International Journal of Public Health, 54*(Suppl 1), 61–67.

Seal, K. H., Bertenthal, D., Maguen, S., Kristian, G., Chu, A., & Marmar, C. R. (2008). Getting beyond "Don't Ask: Don't Tell": An evaluation of U.S. Veterans Administration postdeployment mental health screening of veterans returning from Iraq and Afghanistan. *American Journal of Public Health, 98*(4), 714–720.

Sharkansky, E. J., King, D. W., King, L. A., Wolfe, J., Erikson, D. J., & Stokes, L. R. (2000). Coping with Gulf War combat stress: Mediating and moderating effects. *Journal of Abnormal Psychology, 109*(2), 188–197.

Solomon, Z., Mikulincer, M., & Avitzur, E. (1988). Coping, locus of control, social support, and combat-related posttraumatic stress disorder: A prospective study. *Journal of Personality and Social Psychology, 55*, 279–285.

Spitzer, R. L., Kroenke, K., & Williams, J. B. (1999). Validation and utility of a self-report version of PRIME-MD: The PHQ primary care study. Primary care evaluation of mental disorders. Patient Health Questionnaire. *Journal of the American Medical Association, 282*, 1737–1744.

Tanielian, T., Jaycox, L. H., Schell, T. L., Marshall, G. N., Burnam, M. A., Eibner, C., et al. (2008). *Invisible wounds of war: Summary and recommendations for addressing psychological and cognitive injuries.* Santa Monica, CA: Rand Corporation.

Terhakopian, A., Sinaii, N., Engel, C. C., Schnurr, P. P., & Hoge, C. W. (2008). Estimating population prevalence of posttraumatic stress disorder: An example using the PTSD checklist. *Journal of Traumatic Stress, 21*(3), 290–300.

Toomey, R., Kang, H. K., Karlinsky, J., Baker, D. G., Vasterling, J. J., Alpern, R., et al. (2007). Mental health of U.S. Gulf War veterans 10 years after the war. *British Journal of Psychiatry, 190*, 385–393.

U.S. Army. (2012). *Army 2020: Generating health & discipline in the force.* Washington, DC: Department of the Army.

Vogt, D. S., Pless, A. P., King, L. A., & King, D. W. (2005). Deployment stressors, gender, and mental health outcomes among Gulf War I veterans. *Journal of Traumatic Stress, 18*, 115–127.

Warner, C. H., Appenzeller, G. N., Mullen, K., Warner, C. M., & Grieger, T. A. (2008). Soldier attitudes toward mental health screening and seeking care upon return from combat. *Military Medicine, 173*(6), 563–569.

Warner, C. H., Appenzeller, G. N., Warner, C. M., & Grieger, T. (2009). Psychological effects of deployments on military families. *Psychiatric Annals, 39*(2), 56–63.

Warner, C. M., Warner, C. H., Breitbach, J., Rachal, J., Matuszak, T., & Grieger, T. A. (2007). Depression in entry-level military personnel. *Military Medicine, 172*(8), 795–799.

Wells, T. S., LeardMann, C. A., Fortuna, S. O., Smith, B., Smith, T. C., Ryan, M. A., et al. (2010). A prospective study of depression following combat deployment in support of the wars in Iraq and Afghanistan. *American Journal of Public Health, 100*(1), 90–99.

Williams, J. O., Bell, N. S., & Amorosa, P. J. (2002). Drinking and other risk taking behaviors of enlisted male soldiers in the U.S. Army. *Work, 18*, 141–150.

Wittchen, H. U., Gloster, A., Beesdo, K., Schönfeld, S., & Perkonigg, A. (2009). Posttraumatic stress disorder: Diagnostic and epidemiological perspectives. *CNS Spectrums, 14*(1), 5–12.

Chapter 6
Productivity Loss Associated with Substance Use, Physical Health, and Mental Health

6.1 Overview and Background

As noted in Chap. 4, beginning in 1986 the Department of Defense (DoD) issued a Health Promotion Directive that helps define steps for assuring mission readiness, force health, and fitness of military personnel in an effort to enhance performance. The health promotion directive recognizes and targets behaviors that may interfere with or be detrimental to maximum work productivity. It directed each of the military services to establish health promotion programs that address smoking prevention and cessation, physical fitness, nutrition, stress management, alcohol and drug abuse, and early identification of health problems such as hypertension (DoD Directive 1010.10).

As the military works to maintain force manpower levels through recruitment and retention efforts, it also must consider issues affecting the productivity of service members whose job it is to carry out everyday functions and critical missions. Because the military depends on the productivity of individuals and teams of personnel for successful mission accomplishment, it is critical to understand and minimize factors contributing to productivity loss.

In this chapter, we examine the extent to which work productivity is impacted by substance abuse, physical health problems, and mental health problems. We begin by defining and conceptualizing productivity with a focus on productivity loss. We then examine trends in overall productivity loss as well as trends in productivity loss associated with substance use, physical health, and mental health within the active duty military population from 1995 to 2008. Next, we describe and examine a health and behavioral health model of productivity loss among active duty service members. Productivity loss represents the final outcome of interest noted in Chap. 1 of this book. Our model integrates the key concepts and measures of substance abuse, physical health, and mental health examined in Chaps. 3, 4, and 5 with an emphasis on how they relate and converge to impact productivity among active duty personnel. Our model provides the first assessment of how health and behavioral health factors affect productivity in the military.

R.M. Bray et al., *Understanding Military Workforce Productivity: Effects of Substance Abuse, Health, and Mental Health*, DOI 10.1007/978-0-387-78303-1_6, © Springer Science+Business Media New York 2014

6.1.1   Defining Productivity and Understanding the Impact of Productivity Loss

Productivity is a continually evolving aspect of work performance. According to Riedel, Lynch, Baase, Hymel, and Peterson (2001), the most common measure of worker productivity is absenteeism, which from a broad perspective can be defined as "non-attendance of employees for scheduled work" (Brooke & Price, 1989). However, as these researchers note, simply being at work does not fully reflect the extent to which individuals are productive or at what level they are functioning in terms of particular job requirements. For example, in one study on the contribution of obesity to productivity loss, Ricci and Chee (2005) found that absenteeism alone accounted for only 33 % of the total cost of obesity-related productivity loss. These researchers suggested a multidimensional framework to explain what they term "performance loss," which is the portion of employees' work time that is spent with their energy focused on something other than their job. This framework emphasizes the (a) degree of reduced work capacity, (b) time away from the task, and (c) prevalence within the organization.

This approach offers insights into worker productivity that can be captured concisely by a combination of the terms "absenteeism" and "presenteeism." The latter is an emergent term defined broadly as "the situation when employees are at work but, because of illness, injury, or other conditions, are not functioning at peak levels" (D'Abate & Eddy, 2007). The concept of presenteeism expands the scope of the problem beyond simple absenteeism to encompass the less obvious indicators of diminished productivity, as in the case of a worker who physically comes in to work, but performs below his or her usual level due to personal problems at home or mental health problems such as depression or stress.

Problems related to productivity loss affect organizations at various levels and through various mechanisms. Clearly, productivity loss results in diminished individual performance and work output, which in turn, may reduce intrinsic motivation. In addition, team or group performance may suffer as the result of the reduced performance of one or more individuals as the rest of the team or group struggles to make up the difference. If there is a continuing problem of some team members not pulling their fair share of the load, morale of the team may suffer and conflict and resentment may occur because of the increased work load for some created by others' productivity loss.

These issues exist in the military as well as civilian organizations. Because military units function similar to teams in civilian organizations, they are subject to the same negative consequences arising from worker productivity loss. In fact, such negative consequences may be even more acute in the military because many military personnel lack regular working hours due to the necessity to work until the job is done or until someone relieves them to finish the work (Thomas & Thomas, 1994).

Military systems often do not track absences except in the case of hospitalizations or formal diagnoses of illness or injury, so it is difficult to track productivity loss in terms of absenteeism or presenteeism. Military personnel are expected to operate at full capacity at all times while maintaining optimal levels of physical and mental health. However, threats to these standards abound, especially during periods of increased operational tempo such as those associated with the conflicts in Iraq and Afghanistan (Pinder, Gilbert, Rhodes, Brown, & Bates, 2011). Personal factors, such as substance use, physical health problems, and stress and mental health problems, may negatively impact the productivity levels of affected personnel, which may in turn lead to diminished mission readiness and overall force health. The following sections briefly review the associations of substance use, physical health, and mental health to productivity loss.

6.1.2 Substance Use and Productivity Loss

Research in both civilian and military settings shows clear parallels between substance use and productivity loss. In the past, alcohol-related productivity loss has been estimated at 25 % among civil servants who reported heavy alcohol consumption (GAO, 1970). In a more recent study of civilian workers, 12 % of employees who reported using alcohol reported feeling that their alcohol use had some detrimental effect on their work productivity (Jones, Casswell, & Zhang, 1995). Recent research indicates that DoD wrestles with the same issues in terms of reduced readiness and additional force management costs, in addition to increased medical costs and judicial expenses from alcohol abuse. Indeed it is estimated that alcohol abuse cost DoD $745 million in reduced readiness and judicial expenses (e.g., prosecution of misconduct charges) in 2006 (Harwood, Zhang, Dall, Olaiya, & Fagan, 2009).

Tobacco use also negatively impacts worker productivity. Research suggests that smokers have both increased absenteeism (missing approximately 6.5 more days per year than nonsmokers) and decreased overall workplace productivity (e.g., taking more breaks than nonsmokers) (Halpern, Shikiar, Rentz, & Khan, 2001; MacKenzie, Bartecchi, & Schrier, 1994). Interestingly, this research also reports that former smokers exhibit levels of productivity loss (especially absenteeism) that are between those of smokers and nonsmokers, trending increasingly toward the level of nonsmokers as the length of time following cessation increases (Halpern et al., 2001). Economic analyses have concluded that providing coverage for tobacco cessation programs and other treatments for employees often produce substantial net financial savings through increased productivity, reduced absenteeism, increased health care savings, and reduced life insurance payouts (Agency for Healthcare Research and Quality, 2008).

Illicit drug use has been linked to productivity loss in terms of absenteeism, workplace accidents, and premature mortality. According to the 2008 National Survey on Drug Use and Health (NSDUH), 19.6 % of unemployed adults were current users of illicit drugs, and approximately 8 % of individuals employed full-time and 10.2 % of individuals employed part-time were current users of illicit drugs (Substance Abuse and Mental Health Services Administration, 2009). This translates into approximately 1.8 million unemployed individuals using illicit drugs; and those individuals who are employed but using illicit drugs accrue substantial productivity loss in the form of chronic absenteeism and workplace accidents (Kaestner & Grossman, 1998; U.S. Department of Justice, 2010).

One study of military personnel estimated that lost productivity in the Navy attributed to alcohol and illicit drug use ranged from 9.15 (3.7 %) to 23.12 (9.2 %) annual work days per year (Mehay & Webb, 2007). Based on their analysis of 1999 data, when over 5,000 service members were dismissed from the military due to alcohol and drug violations, the direct cost of this level of productivity loss translated to between $4.4 and $10.9 million, plus an additional $71 million in training and relocation costs to replace personnel in 1 year. Assuming roughly equal separations and costs across all active DoD components, and accounting for inflation from 1999 to 2012, the total for DoD including all service branches balloons to between $24 and $59.4 million per year in lost resources directly related to substance abuse.

6.1.3   Physical Health and Productivity Loss

As noted, losses in productivity can take the form of both absenteeism (employees not coming to work) and presenteeism (employees coming to work but working below their normal level of performance). Some employees may perceive that going to work despite real health problems (such as migraine headaches, back problems, and seasonal allergies) does not constitute a productivity issue; however, the work of employees who "hang in there" and come to work while experiencing health issues does suffer in terms of quantity and quality (Hemp, 2004). For example, Hemp (2004) suggested that painful conditions such as arthritis, headaches, and back problems cost U.S. employers over $47 billion per year in reduced performance. Although different conditions may have different effects on different jobs, they all result in some degree of productivity loss and associated costs to organizations.

In the military environment, Stewart, Ricci, Chee, and Morganstein (2003) illustrated direct costs related to lost productive time for health reasons, including a range of 22 illnesses from the common cold or flu to chronic heart disease. Overall, workers across a variety of standard occupational categories lost an average of 2 h per week due to personal and/or family health reasons. Lost productive time for military personnel was among the lowest of all occupational classifications; however, in terms of absolute resource dollars, the amount remains significant. The 2003 estimates of military health-related lost productive time translate to 2.54 million total lost productive hours per week, or $2.03 billion in lost monetary resources per year ($2.52 billion in 2012 when adjusted for inflation; Friedman, n.d.).

6.1.4   Mental Health and Productivity Loss

Studies have shown that absenteeism declines with successful diagnoses and treatment of some conditions such as depression (e.g., Claxton, Chawla, & Kennedy, 1999).

Therefore, it is important not only to identify the conditions related to diminished productivity but also to understand the ways in which these conditions can be mitigated. Kessler et al. (2006) noted that although absenteeism was higher for workers with bipolar disorders and major depressive disorders than for those with other mood disorders, this was less important than quality of work performance when employees were at work. Individuals with bipolar disorders were absent 22.7 days per year on average, but displayed diminished productivity 35.3 days per year on average. Comparable figures for those with major depressive disorders were 8.7 and 18.2 days, respectively.

Presenteeism has been linked to mental health correlates such as depression. Hemp (2004) cites the cost to organizations of reduced performance attributed to depression as $35 billion per year. Stress has also been shown to be a proximal variable related to productivity loss (Harrison & Martocchio, 1998), although the path of long-term variables to current absenteeism was indirect. The relationship was more fully captured and mediated by both mid-term and short-term variables.

Research shows that mental health issues translate into productivity problems specifically within the military context as well. Hourani, Williams, and Kress (2006) found military personnel with high rates of work and family stress to have higher rates of mental health problems and productivity loss than those with lower stress levels. War exposure in Iraq, Afghanistan, and other locations resulted in posttraumatic stress disorder (PTSD) symptoms and overall poorer health and functioning (Vinokur, Pierce, Lewandowski-Romps, Hobfoll, & Galea, 2011).

6.2 Trends in Productivity Loss

In this section, we examine trends in productivity loss among active duty service members from 1995 to 2008. During this 13-year period each of the DoD Surveys of Health Related Behaviors Among Active Duty Military Personnel (HRB surveys) included the same five items measuring productivity loss described in Chap. 2. These questions were asked without attribution to substance use, physical health, or mental health. To examine trends in productivity loss over time, a composite measure of productivity loss was created for each year of the survey. To create this composite measure, the five items were each dichotomized such that a "No" response indicated that the behavior did not occur in the past 12 months (and was assigned a score of 0), and a "Yes" response indicated that the behavior occurred one or more times in the past 12 months (and was assigned a score of 1). The items were then summed to create a composite measure of productivity loss ranging from 0 to 5. These sum scores were used to estimate and examine an overall trend in productivity loss from 1995 to 2008.

Trends in productivity loss were also examined for selected indicators of substance use (cigarette smoking, heavy drinking, and illicit drug use), physical health (overweight/obesity and exercise), and mental health (depression and stress). These particular indicators were selected to examine trends because they all used the same or comparable definitions and were assessed on each survey from 1995 to 2008. For

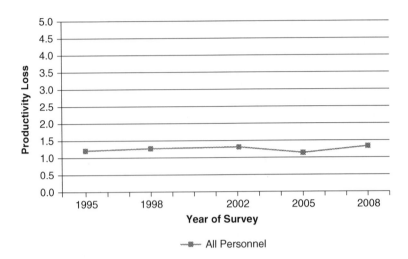

Fig. 6.1 Trends in productivity loss among DoD personnel, 1995–2008

each of these substantive measures, productivity loss scores were computed for each survey year for two different groups using the same approach explained above: (a) those who engaged in the behavior (e.g., were cigarette smokers) or met criteria for the condition (e.g., had high stress) and (b) those who did not engage in the behavior (e.g., were not cigarette smokers) or did not meet the criteria for the condition (e.g., did not have high stress). Examining the productivity loss trend scores for users vs. nonusers permits us to understand the relationship of the three types of behaviors to productivity loss trends over time. We expected that productivity loss would be higher for personnel categorized as "users" or meeting criteria for negative conditions compared to their nonuser counterparts and those not meeting criteria for negative conditions.

6.2.1   Trends in Overall Productivity Loss

Figure 6.1 shows the overall trend in productivity loss from 1995 to 2008. As shown, the overall rate of productivity loss was quite low, beginning with an average score of 1.21 on a 5-point scale in 1995 and increasing slightly, but significantly to a score of 1.33 in 2008 ($\beta=0.004$, $p<0.05$). This suggests that although the active duty population showed generally high rates of productivity over the 13-year period, overall productivity loss has increased. Unfortunately, it is not immediately clear why overall productivity loss increased or whether the increase is of substantive concern, but it may be associated with some aspects of military operations and increased operational tempo with the conflicts in Afghanistan and Iraq. The increases in substance use and mental health problems shown in previous chapters are also hypothesized to be related to increased productivity loss over this period.

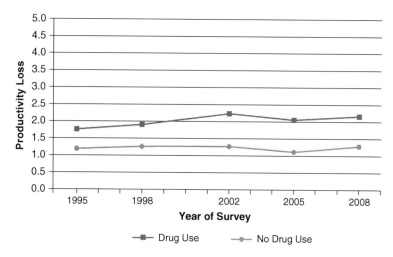

Fig. 6.2 Trends in productivity loss associated with illicit drug use among DoD personnel, 1995–2008

6.2.2   Trends in Productivity Loss by Substance Use

Substance use trends in productivity loss were examined for three indicators of substance use: illicit drug use, heavy alcohol use, and cigarette smoking. Figure 6.2 shows trends in productivity loss by illicit drug use from 1995 to 2008. As expected, illicit drug users consistently reported significantly higher levels of productivity loss than nonusers ($\beta = 0.682$, $p < 0.05$) with the trend lines for users and nonusers being roughly parallel. Although productivity loss generally appears to be rising over time, the change was not statistically significant.

Figure 6.3 shows the trend in productivity loss by heavy alcohol use over time for heavy drinkers and non-heavy drinkers. Heavy drinkers consistently reported significantly higher levels of productivity loss than non-heavy drinkers ($\beta = 0.238$, $p < 0.05$). Levels of productivity loss were relatively flat across the years with some reduction in 2005 but a return to 2002 levels in 2008.

Figure 6.4 shows the trend in productivity loss by cigarette use over time for current smokers and nonsmokers. Across the years cigarette smokers consistently showed significantly higher levels of productivity loss than nonsmokers ($\beta = 0.225$, $p < 0.05$). Similar to the pattern of productivity loss for heavy and non-heavy drinkers, levels of productivity loss for smokers and nonsmokers were also relatively flat over the years with a slight reduction in 2005 followed by an increase in 2008 to the 2002 levels.

When the three substance use indicators are compared across Figs. 6.2, 6.3, 6.4, and 6.5, it is clear that productivity loss among illicit drug users was notably higher than for heavy drinkers or cigarette smokers. Productivity loss for the nonusing groups was about the same for all three measures.

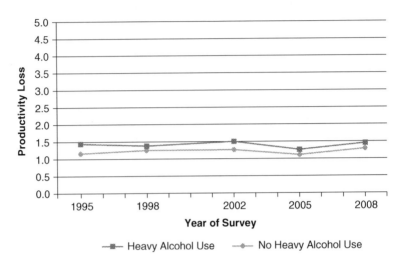

Fig. 6.3 Trends in productivity loss associated with heavy alcohol use among DoD personnel, 1995–2008

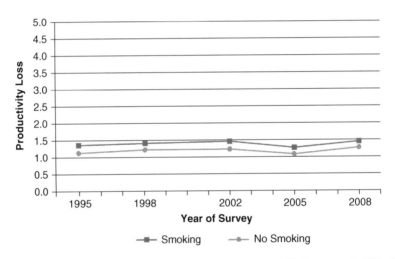

Fig. 6.4 Trends in productivity loss associated with smoking among DoD personnel, 1995–2008

6.2.3   Trends in Productivity Loss by Physical Health

Physical health trends in productivity loss were examined over the 13-year time period using two indices: weight and regular exercise. Figure 6.5 illustrates the trend in regular exercise (defined as moderate or vigorous physical activity at least three times per week) among military personnel. Although overall productivity loss was not significantly different over time by exercise level, personnel who did not exercise regularly consistently reported significantly more productivity loss than

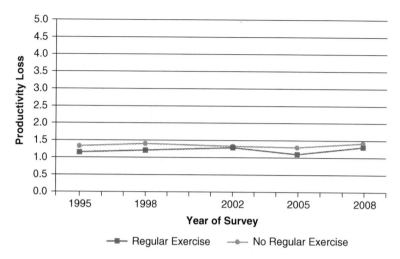

Fig. 6.5 Trends in productivity loss associated with exercise among DoD personnel, 1995–2008

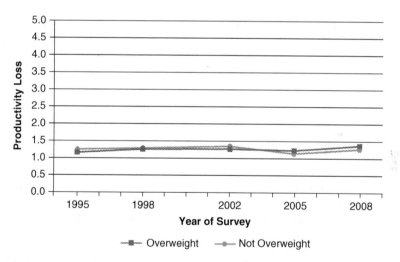

Fig. 6.6 Trends in productivity loss associated with overweight among DoD personnel, 1995–2008

personnel who reported exercising regularly ($\beta = -0.175$, $p < 0.05$) although the magnitude of these differences was rather small.

Productivity loss trends were also examined by weight status, specifically "overweight" and "not overweight" status as measured by the body mass index (BMI). As shown in Fig. 6.6, differences between the two groups were quite small, but during the latter part of the period, overweight personnel showed higher rates of productivity loss than their nonoverweight counterparts. The overall trend was quite flat over the 13-year time frame.

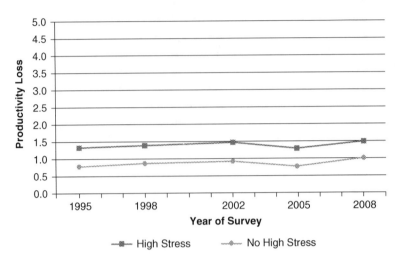

Fig. 6.7 Trends in productivity loss associated with stress among DoD personnel, 1995–2008

Taken together, Figs. 6.5 and 6.6 indicate that personnel who engage in more negative physical health behaviors (i.e., not maintaining a healthy weight or exercising regularly) were more likely to report productivity loss than personnel who engage in healthier behaviors although these differences were small and less pronounced for weight.

6.2.4   Trends in Productivity Loss by Mental Health

Mental health trends in productivity loss were examined over time for two measures: stress and depression. Figure 6.7 shows the trend in productivity loss associated with stress among military personnel. As shown, personnel who reported high levels of stress consistently showed significantly greater productivity loss than personnel who did not report high levels of stress ($\beta=0.555$, $p<0.05$). Interestingly, productivity loss increased significantly over time both for those reporting high stress ($\beta=0.008$, $p<0.05$) and for those not reporting high stress ($\beta=0.012$, $p<0.05$); this suggests that even low to moderate stress can reduce productivity among military personnel.

Figure 6.8 illustrates the trend in productivity loss by depression symptoms. Overall, there is a clear pattern of higher productivity loss among personnel who reported symptoms of depression than among personnel who did not report symptoms of depression ($\beta=0.556$, $p<0.05$). Similarly, there was a significant increase in productivity loss across the years among personnel who reported symptoms of depression ($\beta=0.008$, $p<0.05$), but no increase in productivity loss among personnel who did not report such symptoms.

Together, Figs. 6.7 and 6.8 show that personnel who reported experiencing mental health problems were more likely to report productivity loss than personnel who did not report such problems.

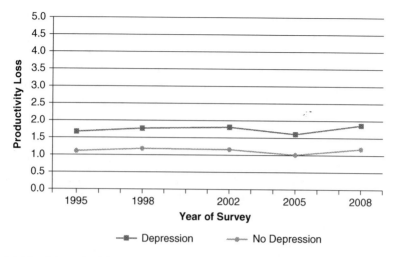

Fig. 6.8 Trends in productivity loss associated with depression among DoD personnel, 1995–2008

6.3 A Health and Behavioral Health Model of Productivity Loss

Previous research and our findings suggest that substance use, physical health, and mental health factors may be related to productivity loss among active duty military personnel. These correlates point to possible prevention and intervention points; however, to formulate the most effective and impactful action plan for addressing these issues, it is important to understand how substance use, physical health, and mental health components relate to one another as well as to productivity loss. To this end, using the constructs discussed earlier, we developed and estimated a health and behavioral health model of productivity loss that includes the various substance use, physical health, and mental health indicators as predictors. This model synthesizes findings from previous chapters and extends them to a broader framework of personnel productivity and readiness. Understanding the determinants of productivity and the magnitude of their effects will yield information that can then be translated into policy and procedures to reduce productivity losses, thereby increasing overall force readiness and health.

6.3.1 Model Constructs and Latent Factors

Model estimation was performed in two stages. In the first stage, latent measurement factors were evaluated for the domains of substance abuse, mental health, and productivity loss. Indicators of substance abuse and mental health were based on the outcome measures from the previous chapters. More specifically, indicators for the substance use latent factor were alcohol dependence, one or more serious consequences of alcohol use, nicotine dependence, heavy drinking, past month smoking, and past month illicit drug use. Indicators for the mental health latent factor were PTSD, depression, generalized anxiety disorder, significant work or family stress, receipt of mental health counseling services, and past year suicidal ideation. A physical health latent factor was not used because there were only three indicators (overweight/obese, illness in the past year, and injury in the past year), resulting in a measurement model that could not be independently evaluated for fit.[1] Estimating this physical health factor jointly with each of the other measurement models indicated that the three physical health items did not load well on a latent factor.

The five items used to measure productivity loss noted earlier in the chapter were also used to form a latent factor as the main outcome measure for the model. These items examined the number of work days in the past year that service members indicated that they (a) worked below their normal level of performance; (b) were hurt in an on-the-job accident; (c) left work early for a reason other than an errand or early holiday leave; (d) were late for work by 30 min or more; or (e) did not come to work at all because of an illness or personal accident.

Each measurement model was estimated with confirmatory factor analysis (CFA) in Mplus version 6 (Muthén & Muthén, 1998–2010) and evaluated for fit using two fit indices: the comparative fit index (CFI) and root-mean-square error of approximation (RMSEA). Generally acceptable cutoffs for these indexes are 0.95 and higher for the CFI and 0.06 or lower for the RMSEA (Hu & Bentler, 1999). Fit for each of the latent factors was good, indicating that the dimensions of substance use, mental health, and productivity loss could be represented in the overall model by these latent factors instead of the larger number of individual component items.

Figure 6.9 and Table 6.1 summarize the standardized factor loadings and fit indices for the substance use, mental health, and productivity loss latent factors.

6.3.2   *Estimating Productivity Loss*

The second stage of estimating the theoretical model of productivity loss was to enter the substance use and mental health latent factors into a path model along with other constructs representing physical health (overweight or obesity, illness in the past year, injury in the past year) and activity limitations due to physical or mental health problems. Paths were included to estimate the direct impact of substance use, mental health, and the three physical health items on productivity loss, as well as indirect pathways from these predictors through physical health- and mental health-related activity limitations.

---

[1]The physical health latent factor did not work well; therefore, this factor was not included as a composite measure.

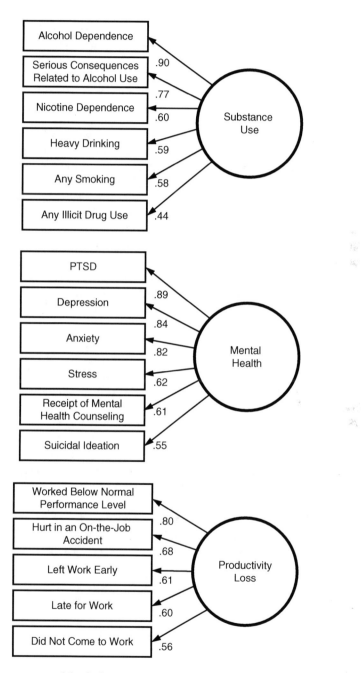

Fig. 6.9 Measurement models of substance use, mental health, and productivity loss among DoD personnel, 2008

Table 6.1 Fit indices for the substance use, mental health, and productivity loss latent factors

Factors	CFI	RMSEA index
Substance use	0.922	0.041
Mental health	0.994	0.019
Productivity loss	0.970	0.031

Figure 6.10 presents the path estimates (as standardized regression coefficients) for significant predictive paths (at $p < 0.05$ or less) in the model. The latent factors for substance use, mental health, and productivity loss are represented by circles, whereas the observed or manifest variables of overweight/obesity, past year illness, past year injury, physical health-limited usual activities, and mental health-limited usual activities are represented by boxes.

As shown in Fig. 6.10, the strongest predictor (gauged by the magnitude of the standardized path coefficient) was physical health-related activity limitations ($\beta = 0.24$, $p < 0.001$). Mental health was also strongly predictive of productivity loss, with a standardized regression coefficient of 0.21 ($p < 0.001$) for the latent factor measuring mental health problems. Injury and illness were also predictive of increased productivity loss ($\beta = 0.17$, $p < 0.001$; $\beta = 0.11$, $p < 0.001$, respectively). Mental health-related activity limitations and substance use were not as strongly related to productivity loss, although both were still significant predictors of productivity loss ($\beta = 0.09$, $p < 0.001$; $\beta = 0.08$, $p < 0.001$, respectively).

Indirect or mediated effects of substance use, physical health, and mental health predictors on productivity loss were tested with Wald confidence intervals around the estimated mediated effect. Estimates of mediated effects were formed as the product of the path from a predictor to the intermediate variable (mental or physical health limitations in this model) and the path from the intermediate variable to productivity loss (MacKinnon, 2008). The majority of indirect effects were significant. Specifically, higher scores on the mental health latent factor (i.e., greater mental health problems) as well as having an injury or illness in the past year were associated with increased likelihood of both physical health- and mental health-related activity limitations; both types of limitations were positively associated with increased productivity loss. Indirect effects that were not significant were those from substance use through physical health- and mental health-related activity limitations, and the indirect effect from overweight to productivity loss through physical health limitations.

6.4   Summary and Discussion

6.4.1   Trends

Overall productivity loss among military personnel was relatively low across the 13-year period from 1995 to 2008, reflecting the success of the military in accomplishing its evolving missions over time. Although low, overall productivity loss

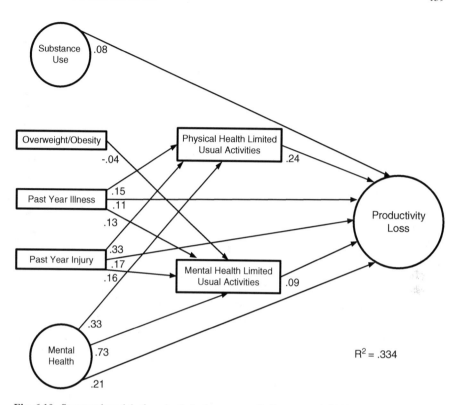

Fig. 6.10 Structural model of productivity loss among DoD personnel, 2008

increased slightly but significantly from 1995 to 2008, suggesting that the military may be beginning to face problems with productivity at a time when operational tempo has been at its highest level in decades. Specifically, productivity loss showed an increasing trend from 1995 to 2008 among personnel who reported having high stress and symptoms of depression. Both of these issues are likely impacted by increased operational tempo. Alternative pathways to reducing service member mental health burdens should continue to be explored.

Most notably, when we compared productivity loss across the survey years, we found that service members who engaged in substance use or who had physical health problems or mental health problems had higher levels of productivity loss than personnel who did not report substance use or experience physical or mental health problems. Specifically, personnel who reported illicit drug use, heavy alcohol use, cigarette smoking, high stress, being overweight, and having symptoms of depression showed higher levels of productivity loss than personnel who did not report these behaviors. Productivity loss was also higher among personnel who did not exercise regularly compared to those who engaged in regular exercise. These findings add a new dimension to the literature surrounding each of these factors and their isolated impact on overall health and well-being. In particular, within the military community, when one or more of these factors converge to reduce productivity, the success of the military mission may be negatively affected. In addition, due to the team-based nature of many military operations, losses in individual productivity are likely to impact overall team performance, cohesion, and morale.

However, this team-oriented structure also represents an opportunity for prevention and intervention efforts through the social support channels built into the team itself. Keeping team members engaged with one another and with their job assignments may serve a preventive function by protecting against the development of substance use, physical health, mental health, and productivity problems. Team members may also be effective in reaching and helping individuals who are already affected by these problems.

6.4.2   Productivity Loss Model

The goal of our productivity loss model was to provide a succinct picture of the relationships and of the predictive power of the large number of substance use, physical health, and mental health variables that we examined in prior chapters on productivity loss. Our approach to simplifying this set of variables was to develop substance use and mental health latent factors using the key outcome indicators for these constructs. Our factor analyses showed that the substance use outcomes (alcohol dependence, serious consequences related to alcohol use, nicotine dependence, heavy drinking, any cigarette smoking, and any illicit drug use) and the mental health outcomes (PTSD, depression, anxiety, stress, receipt of mental health counseling, and suicidal ideation) clustered together nicely to form good-fitting latent factors. Similarly, the five items measuring productivity loss (worked below normal performance level, hurt in an on-the-job accident, left work early, late for work, or did not come to work) also clustered together to form a single factor that served as the overall outcome measure in the model.

The substance use and mental health constructs coupled with our other measures of overweight/obesity, past year illness, past year injury, physical health-limited usual activities, and mental health-limited usual activities did a good job of predicting productivity loss. The model had an overall R^2 of 0.334, which is relatively strong in a complex behavioral study such as this one.

As we saw in our structural model (Fig. 6.10), some variables had direct effects on productivity loss, some had indirect effects, and some had both direct and indirect effects. The variables with the strongest direct effects were physical health-limited usual activities, mental health, and past year injury. These findings also have strong face validity and indicate that service members who have physical health limitations, who have mental health problems, and who have been injured are less able to be effective in their jobs and hence have higher rates of productivity loss. This is consistent with other research showing that among both active duty and Reserve component personnel, service members with high stress and other mental health problems, as well physical illness and injury, had greater productivity loss than those without these problems (Bray et al., 2009; Hourani et al., 2006, 2007). Considering the immediate impacts of these factors on productivity, we believe that long-term consequences may also exist in terms of impacts on overall force readiness due to attrition of service members who do not seek help for these issues.

The other variables showing direct effects on productivity loss were past year illness, mental health-limited usual activities, and substance use. Service members who are ill or not able to function well because of mental health limitations are less able to carry out their normal duties. Similarly, those who engage in substance use may have increased illness or may experience hangovers or negative consequences such that they are not able to function at normal levels and their productivity is diminished. In line with this, Mattiko, Rae Olmsted, Brown, and Bray (2011) found that heavy alcohol users showed nearly three times the rate of self-reported serious consequences and over twice the rate of self-reported productivity loss compared to moderate/heavy drinkers. These findings suggest that there may be a qualitative shift in drinking problems as the levels of consumption increase.

Of note is the finding that even when accounting for physical health- and mental health-related activity limitations, substance use and mental health problems were still uniquely predictive of productivity loss. This suggests that mental health and substance use have a unique harmful impact on service members' productivity that does not also result in more serious or long-term limitations in daily functioning. However, both types of activity limitation were strongly predicted by the mental health factor and illness or injury in the past year, indicating that productivity loss may also arise from these predictors, causing more serious disruptions in daily functioning.

Substance use was unique in the model in that it had a direct effect only on productivity loss and did not show a significant association with any other variables in the model. Further, even though these substance use results were statistically significant, they were only of moderate strength. This is somewhat surprising in view of the known problems that often result from excessive alcohol use and illicit drug use (Halpern et al., 2001; Harwood et al., 2009; Kaestner & Grossman, 1998; MacKenzie et al., 1994; U.S. Department of Justice, 2010). Two possible explanations are that (a) personnel who use illicit drugs or drink heavily do so at times when they are not working so the effects typically do not decrease work performance or (b) if they use during times that may affect them at work (e.g., hangovers from a prior night's drinking), they are able to cover up many of their problems and still perform their work at a relatively adequate level. Substance use was not predictive of either type of activity limitation, suggesting that any loss in productivity is a direct consequence of use not associated with any longer-term or more serious activity limitations. These findings suggest that negative consequences associated with substance use may have a short, and perhaps an intense, impact on behaviors (i.e., a temporary high from drug use or a hangover from heavy drinking) that have a more limited impact on productivity loss.

In addition to its direct effect on productivity loss, mental health also had a strong indirect effect on productivity loss through the two indicators of limited activities: (a) mental health-limited usual activities ($\beta=0.73$, $p<0.05$) and (b) physical health-limited usual activities ($\beta = 0.33$, $p < 0.05$). It is expected that mental health problems would be positively associated with mental health-limited usual activities, but less expected that mental health problems would be a strong predictor of physical health limitations. The latter finding may partially reflect some of the correlational properties of the data (i.e., that physical activity limitations may also predict mental health problems such as depression). It may also underscore the broad impact of mental health problems that can result in limitations on mental and physical activities.

A corollary and important implication from these paths in the model is that if we can find ways to improve mental health and to reduce injury, illness, and substance use, we should also see improvements in productivity (i.e., reduced productivity loss) and ultimately increased readiness. Personnel with good mental health are more likely to be more effective and efficient at work and to be fully present and engaged in productive work (D'Abate & Eddy, 2007). Additionally, although rates of productivity loss have been relatively low and the trends we examined showed only small increases over time (i.e., productivity loss increased, meaning productivity declined), the practical implications for DoD resources can be highly significant in terms of monetary losses and reductions in morale and overall readiness. Bliese, Adler, and Castro (2011) pointed out that small and sometimes nonsignificant effects in a single study (e.g., in preventative mental health programs geared to teach resilience skills) can have practical significance and become important over the longer term when the cumulative impact is realized. A similar point can be made for the cumulative economic savings and readiness improvements that can be realized from even small reductions in productivity loss.

We recognize that our findings are limited by the cross-sectional nature of the HRB survey data, which preclude definitive causal statements about the relationships detailed in our model of productivity loss. To address this, variables were selected to minimize the likelihood of causal paths actually being the reverse of how they were specified in the model. For example, it is unlikely that any of the indicators of productivity loss caused physical health- or mental health-related activity limitations. Similarly, it is much more feasible that a significant illness or injury caused activity limitations (and also productivity loss) rather than the reverse. The greatest equivocation in path directionality is likely from mental health to activity limitations and productivity loss. There is evidence suggesting that mental health problems can negatively affect activity and hence productivity (Gordon, Ganesan, Towell, & Kirkham, 2002; Tanielian & Jaycox, 2008), but other data suggest that chronic illness and limitations to one's daily routine can affect mental health negatively (World Federation for Mental Health, 2010).

6.5   Recap

Our model of productivity loss indicates that military work effectiveness is inversely related to substance abuse, physical health, and mental health factors. Higher rates of these types of problems were associated with reduced productivity and lowered military readiness. Physical health limitations, mental health problems, past year injury, and past year illness were the factors with the largest impact on productivity loss. Substance use still played a significant role, but was less important in explaining productivity loss, perhaps because negative consequences from substance use (especially short-term excessive drinking) are more short-lived and can be recovered from reasonably quickly compared to mental health problems, illness and injury, and physical health and mental health limitations. Our findings have implications for monitoring productivity loss as well as developing job-specific productivity measures within the military.

References

Agency for Healthcare Research and Quality. (2008). *Systems change: Treating tobacco use and dependence*. Retrieved October 11, 2012, from http://www.ahrq.gov/clinic/tobacco/systems.htm

Bliese, P. D., Adler, A. B., & Castro, C. A. (2011). Research-based preventive mental health care strategies in the military. In A. B. Adler, P. D. Bliese, & C. A. Castro (Eds.), *Deployment psychology: Evidence-based strategies to promote mental health in the military* (pp. 103–124). Washington, DC: American Psychological Association.

Bray, R. M., Pemberton, M. R., Hourani, L. L., Witt, M., Rae Olmsted, K. L., Brown, J. M., et al. (2009). *2008 Department of defense survey of health related behaviors among active duty military personnel*. Report prepared for TRICARE Management Activity, Office of the Assistant Secretary of Defense (Health Affairs) and U.S. Coast Guard. Research Triangle Park, NC: Research Triangle Institute.

Brooke, P. P., & Price, J. L. (1989). The determinants of employee absenteeism: An empirical test of a causal model. *Journal of Occupational Psychology, 62*, 1–19.

Claxton, A. J., Chawla, A. J., & Kennedy, S. (1999). Absenteeism among employees treated for depression. *Journal of Occupational and Environmental Medicine, 41*, 605–611.

D'Abate, C. P., & Eddy, E. R. (2007). Engaging in personal business on the job: Extending the presenteeism construct. *Human Resource Development Quarterly, 18*(3), 361–383.

Department of Defense. (1986, March 11). *Directive No. 1010.10. Health promotion*. Washington, DC: U.S. Department of Defense.

Friedman, S. M. (n.d.) *The inflation calculator*. Retrieved June 4, 2013, from http://www.westegg.com/inflation/

General Accounting Office. (1970). *Comptroller general's report to subcommittee on alcoholism and narcotics*. Washington, DC: Government Printing Office.

Gordon, A. L., Ganesan, V., Towell, A., & Kirkham, F. J. (2002). Functional outcome following stroke in children. *Journal of Child Neurology, 17*, 429–434.

Halpern, M. T., Shikiar, R., Rentz, A. M., & Khan, Z. M. (2001). Impact of smoking status on workplace absenteeism and productivity. *Tobacco Control, 10*, 233–238.

Harrison, D. A., & Martocchio, J. J. (1998). Time for absenteeism: A 20-year review of origins, offshoots, and outcomes. *Journal of Management, 24*(3), 305–350.

Harwood, H. J., Zhang, Y., Dall, T. M., Olaiya, S. T., & Fagan, N. K. (2009). Economic implications of reduced binge drinking among the military health system's TRICARE Prime plan beneficiaries. *Military Medicine, 174*, 728–736.

Hemp, P. (2004). Presenteeism: At work—But out of it. *Harvard Business Review, 82*(49–58), 155.

Hourani, L. L., Bray, R. M., Marsden, M. E., Witt, M., Vandermaas-Peeler, R., Scheffler, S., et al. (2007). *2006 Department of defense survey of health related behaviors among the guard and reserve force* (Technical Report No. RTI/9842/001/201-FR). Research Triangle Park, NC: Research Triangle Institute.

Hourani, L. L., Williams, T. V., & Kress, A. M. (2006). Stress, mental health, and job performance among active duty military personnel: Findings from the 2002 Department of Defense Health-Related Behaviors Survey. *Military Medicine, 171*, 849–856.

Hu, L., & Bentler, P. M. (1999). Cutoff criteria for fit indexes in covariance structure analysis: Conventional criteria versus new alternatives. *Structural Equation Modeling, 6*, 1–55.

Jones, S., Casswell, S., & Zhang, J. F. (1995). The economic costs of alcohol-related absenteeism and reduced productivity among the working population of New Zealand. *Addiction, 90*, 1455–1461.

Kaestner, R., & Grossman, M. (1998). The effect of drug use on workplace accidents. *Labour Economics, 5*, 267–294.

Kessler, R. C., Akiskal, H. S., Ames, M., Birnbaum, H., Greenberg, P., Hirschfeld, R. M., et al. (2006). Prevalence and effects of mood disorders on work performance in a nationally representative sample of U. S. workers. *American Journal of Psychiatry, 163*, 1561–1568.

MacKenzie, T. D., Bartecchi, C. E., & Schrier, R. W. (1994). The human costs of tobacco use (2). *New England Journal of Medicine, 330*, 975–980.

MacKinnon, D. P. (2008). *Introduction to statistical mediation analysis*. Mahwah, NJ: Erlbaum.

Mattiko, M., Rae Olmsted, K., Brown, J. M., & Bray, R. M. (2011). Alcohol use and negative consequences among active duty military personnel. *Addictive Behaviors, 36*, 608–614.

Mehay, S., & Webb, N. J. (2007). Workplace drug prevention programs: Does zero tolerance work? *Applied Economics, 39*, 2743–2751.

Muthén, L. K., & Muthén, B. O. (1998–2010). *Mplus user's guide* (6th ed). Los Angeles, CA: Muthén & Muthén.

Pinder, E., Gilbert, A., Rhodes, J., Brown, D., & Bates, M. (2011). *Worksite health promotion: Wellness in the workplace*. Silver Spring, MD: Defense Centers of Excellence for Psychological Health and Traumatic Brain Injury.

Ricci, J. A., & Chee, E. (2005). Lost productive time associated with excess weight in the U.S. workforce. *Journal of Occupational and Environmental Medicine, 47*(12), 1227–1234.

Riedel, J. E., Lynch, W., Baase, C., Hymel, P., & Peterson, K. W. (2001). The effect of disease prevention and health promotion on workplace productivity: A literature review. *American Journal of Health Promotion, 15*, 167–191.

Stewart, W. F., Ricci, J. A., Chee, E., & Morganstein, D. (2003). Lost productive work time costs from health conditions in the United States: Results from the American Productivity Audit. *Journal of Occupational and Environmental Medicine, 45*(12), 1234–1246.

Substance Abuse and Mental Health Services Administration. (2009). *Results from the 2008 National Survey on Drug Use and Health: National Findings* (Office of Applied Studies, NSDUH Series H-36, HHS Publication No. SMA 09-4434). Rockville, MD.

Tanielian, T., & Jaycox, L. (Eds.). (2008). *Invisible wounds of war: Psychological and cognitive injuries, their consequences, and services to assist recovery*. Santa Monica, CA: RAND Corporation, MG-720-CCF.

Thomas, P. J., & Thomas, M. D. (1994). Effects of sex, marital status, and parental status on absenteeism among Navy personnel. *Military Psychology, 6*(2), 95–108.

U.S. Department of Justice. (2010). *National Drug Threat Assessment 2010*. Johnstown, PA: National Drug Intelligence Center.

Vinokur, A. D., Pierce, P. F., Lewandowski-Romps, L., Hobfoll, S. E., & Galea, S. (2011). Effects of war exposure on air force personnel's mental health, job burnout and other organizational related outcomes. *Journal of Occupational Health Psychology, 16*(1), 3–17.

World Federation for Mental Health. (2010). *Mental health and chronic physical illnesses: The need for continued and integrated care*. Retrieved June 14, 2013, from http://www.wfmh.org/2010DOCS/WMHDAY2010.pdf

Chapter 7
Summary and Implications of Findings

7.1 Overview and Background

The physical and mental health of the active duty military force is critical to the military's mission of maintaining national security and supporting peacetime operations. A healthy and well-functioning force will be able to sustain a high degree of productivity and readiness to defend our interests across the world. Military fitness training is among the most rigorous of any occupation, and the majority of personnel are fit, healthy, and resilient; however, during the era of Operation Iraqi Freedom (OIF), 2003–2011, and Operation Enduring Freedom (OEF), (2001 to present) the challenges of maintaining a healthy force have been magnified by years of war and multiple deployments with their attendant challenges. Indeed, these conflicts have given rise to broader, more holistic conceptualizations of fitness with the most comprehensive called Total Force Fitness, an approach that recognizes and encompasses the complexity of human behavior. The new Total Force Fitness paradigm incorporates components of both mind and body and proposes eight cross-cutting domains of fitness: behavioral, social, physical, environmental, medical, spiritual, nutritional, and psychological (Jonas et al., 2010). This new fitness paradigm accounts for the increased complexity of the military mission and acknowledges that the paradigm based primarily around physical fitness is inadequate to address the broad array of challenges and cross-cutting skills needed by military personnel to be fully productive.

Even though we were not able to consider the integration of all of these domains, the analyses in this book provide a key step in addressing the overlap in physical, behavioral, and psychological aspects of fitness and their relationship to productivity. Many of the analyses in this book focus on events in 2008 (the most recent year of HRB data analyzed) which was during the midst of the OIF/OEF conflicts. Even though OIF has officially concluded and OEF is beginning to wind down, many of the substance abuse, physical health, and mental health concerns that emerged during the height and intensity of these conflicts are continuing issues for the military. The costs of substance abuse, poor physical health, and mental health problems—whether they are monetary, legal, and/or personal/family-related—compromise

R.M. Bray et al., *Understanding Military Workforce Productivity: Effects of Substance Abuse, Health, and Mental Health*, DOI 10.1007/978-0-387-78303-1_7,
© Springer Science+Business Media New York 2014

our military's ability to protect the nation in the most effective, efficient manner. For example, it has been estimated that 55–95 % of the total costs of major depression and posttraumatic stress disorder (PTSD) alone can be attributed to reduced productivity (Tanielian & Jaycox, 2008).

The active duty military population is relatively young (see Chap. 2) and has been judged to have better physical health than the U.S. general population (Smith et al., 2007). The wellness and readiness of the military in all branches has been a key focus of policymakers, service providers, and researchers, particularly in recent years. The military has taken the lead in funneling large amounts of resources toward expanding and improving health and mental health services for military personnel returning from war; developing innovative technologies to address the physical injuries of wounded warriors; funding cutting-edge research in the form of treatment, intervention, and prevention studies of psychological and cognitive injuries such as PTSD, traumatic brain injury (TBI), and suicide; and promoting resilience and anti-stigma efforts (Meredith et al., 2011).

Despite this commendable work and associated advancements, there are many remaining issues of concern. These include leading a force that has been at war for over 10 years and has personnel and families affected by combat-related wounds, other injuries and illnesses, stress related to high operational tempo and repeated deployments, and even preservice health conditions (Department of the Army, 2012b). Indeed, a recent Institute of Medicine (IOM) report concluded that veterans, service members and their families face complex health, economic, and social readjustment issues and challenges as they return home from the OIF/OEF conflicts and that the magnitude of these problems will require considerable additional sustained effort (IOM, 2013). Some of the specific challenges currently facing military leaders and policymakers include simultaneously addressing the comorbidity of physical and behavioral health issues; managing prescription medications to provide needed relief from pain and suffering while avoiding drug and alcohol misuse, abuse, and addiction; preventing and treating substance abuse problems and disorders; preventing and treating complex mental health issues such as PTSD, TBI, and suicidal ideation; and reducing the stigma associated with seeking and receiving care (Department of the Army, 2012b; IOM, 2012, 2013).

Physical and psychological demands have been intense during OIF/OEF for military personnel whose ability to perform at high levels to defend our interests across the world is critical. Physical and behavioral health considerations are among the most important factors influencing military productivity and readiness. The OIF/OEF period of war and strife has propelled the physical and behavioral health issues of the military into the spotlight and media attention has often raised important questions with no ready answers or solutions. To address health and readiness issues effectively—particularly those related to operational stress, combat, and trauma—information about problem rates and effective treatments and interventions is needed to guide action. Without question, the better the information, the more complete and informative the answers and solutions that can be proffered. The intent of this book is to provide this information in a consolidated and digestible format; the intent of this chapter is to summarize key findings and implications for actionable ways forward.

7.2 Key Findings and Implications

7.2.1 Substance Abuse

Findings from Chap. 3 showed a dramatic decline in illicit drug use from 1980 to 2002 accompanied by increases from 2002 to 2008, long-term declines in cigarette use; and a greater stability in heavy drinking among active duty personnel. Illicit drug abuse includes illegal or street drugs such as marijuana, heroin, and cocaine, as well as the nonmedical use of prescription-type amphetamines/stimulants, tranquilizers/muscle relaxers, barbiturates/sedatives, and pain relievers, In 2008, during the month prior to taking the survey, 12 % of military personnel reported using illicit drugs, 47 % reported binge drinking, 20 % reported engaging in heavy drinking, and 31 % reported smoking cigarettes.

Increases in illicit drug use from 2002 to 2008 were driven by increases in nonmedical use of prescription drugs, notably pain relievers, perhaps to ease pain related to high rates of injury among military personnel (Bray, Rae Olmsted, & Williams, 2012). Misuse of prescription drugs, or nonmedical use of these drugs, increased from 2 % in 2002 to 11 % in 2008, while rates of illicit drug use excluding prescription drug misuse, continued at the low rates observed in 2002 around 2 %. It is important to recall from Chap. 3 that in 2005 and 2008, questionnaire changes in the HRB survey rendered the findings on illicit drug use not *directly* comparable to prior years, though we believe that the questionnaire changes improved our ability to capture more specific information and therefore improved our reporting capabilities. In the 2005 HRB survey, examples of specific types of illicit drugs were added for clarity; in 2008, questions about illegal drugs and prescription drugs were asked separately, and questions about "analgesics" were changed to "pain relievers" to reduce ambiguity for survey respondents. The result may have been an increase in the measured prevalence of illicit drugs overall in 2005 and 2008 and in the use of specific classes of illicit drugs, notably, prescription drugs used for nonmedical purposes. It should be further noted that misuse of prescription drugs to relieve pain suggests a very different motivation for use than the motivation of getting "high" typically associated with illicit drug use. More research is needed to understand the intent and differing motivations for these uses.

Heavy drinking was relatively stable over time, but showed gradual increases from 1998 to 2008 (15–20 %), consistent with increases in binge drinking during the same period (35–47 %). The percentage of military personnel reporting serious consequences related to alcohol use declined from 1980 to 1998, but increased to 2008. Alcohol dependence decreased in recent years, and nicotine dependence remained stable.

Overall, after adjusting for population demographic differences, the rate of illicit drug use was lower among military personnel than among civilians, whereas the rates of heavy drinking and binge drinking were higher among military personnel than civilians. The overall rate of cigarette use was similar between the two populations. Military and civilian differences in substance use varied by age group, however, with rates of illicit drug use (including prescription misuse) being greater among older military personnel than civilians, rates of heavy and binge drinking being higher among younger military personnel than civilians, and smoking being lower among older military personnel than civilians. These differences may reflect cohort differences or the effects of military policies designed to combat use of these substances.

Our modeling analyses showed a number of significant predictors for illicit drug use, heavy alcohol use, and cigarette use. Screening positive for PTSD, heavy drinking, illness, injury, risk-taking, and junior pay grade were among the stronger predictors of illicit drug use. Those screening positive for PTSD were 1.75 times more likely than those not screening positive to have used illicit drugs in the past month. Service members in pay grades E1–E3 were 1.64 times more likely those in pay grades O4–O10 to have used illicit drugs in the past month and heavy drinkers were 1.63 times more likely than those who were not heavy drinkers to have used illicit drugs in the past month. Analyses for heavy drinking showed that gender, cigarette smoking, and age were among the strongest predictors. Men were 2.78 times more than women to be heavy drinkers, smokers were 2.54 times more likely than nonsmokers to be heavy drinkers, and persons aged 21–25 were 2.20 times more likely than persons aged 35 or older to be heavy drinkers. Finally, analyses of cigarette smoking found that pay grade and heavy drinking were the strongest predictors. Personnel in pay grades E1–E3 were 9.38 times more likely, those in pay grades E4–E6 were 6.97 times more likely, and those in pay grades E7–E9 were 4.23 times more likely to smoke cigarettes compared with those in pay grades O4–O10. Heavy drinkers were 2.52 times more likely to smoke than non-heavy drinkers.

Considering all predictors together, age and pay grade were among the strongest predictors of use of illicit drugs, alcohol, or cigarettes. Use was more common among junior enlisted personnel and younger personnel. Use of any of the three substances was also related to using other substances, deployment that included moderate or high combat exposure, and to risk-taking. Screening positive for PTSD was also a significant predictor of illicit drug use and heavy drinking. Significant predictors of heavy drinking and cigarette use included high work or family stress; and a significant predictor of cigarette use was screening positive for depression. Consequences related to substance use were also associated with risk-taking, but were not associated with deployment or combat exposure. Those screening positive for PTSD were more likely to report serious consequences related to alcohol use and alcohol dependence, and those screening positive for depression were more likely to be nicotine-dependent. These findings point to the comorbid relationship of substance use, stress, and mental health problems. They also offer support for the self-medication hypothesis that service members experiencing stress or mental health problems may be turning to substance use as a possible way of coping with these problems (Harris & Edlund, 2005).

Excessive alcohol use in the form of heavy and binge drinking is the most serious substance abuse problem facing the military and is related to a military culture that supports and facilitates it (Ames, Cunradi, Moore, & Stern, 2007; Bray, Brown, & Williams, 2013; Bray et al., 2009, 2010). Heavy drinking is of particular concern because it is related to engaging in other high-risk behaviors such as wearing seatbelts less frequently, driving over the speed limit, and smoking more than half a pack of cigarettes a day (Williams, Bell, & Amoroso, 2002). New onset of heavy drinking, binge drinking, and alcohol-related problems is also related to combat exposure (Jacobson et al., 2008).

A 2012 IOM committee conducted a comprehensive, in-depth review of substance use in the military including problem rates, and approaches to prevention, screening, diagnosis, and treatment of substance use disorders. The committee reached the distressing conclusion that "alcohol and other drug use in the armed forces remain unacceptably high, constitute a public health crisis, and both are detrimental to force readiness and psychological fitness" (IOM, 2012). To address these issues the committee asserts that the "highest levels of military leadership must acknowledge these alarming facts and combat them using an arsenal of public health strategies, including proactively attacking substance use problems before they begin by limiting access to certain medications and alcohol" (IOM, 2012). Clearly, there are numerous challenges facing military leaders, policymakers, and researchers to address these substance use concerns. The HRB surveys have been a key tool in tracking and monitoring substance use rates and consequences to provide military leaders with much of the information they need to understand where progress is being made and where problems and challenges remain.

7.2.2 Health and Health Behaviors

Chapter 4 examined healthy lifestyles and health promotion with an emphasis on overweight and obesity status, injury, and illness. It also examined the health-related behaviors of active duty military personnel using selected criteria set by the *Healthy People 2010* initiative. Of the nine *Healthy People 2010* objectives examined, service members met or exceeded only the objectives for exercise and obesity. The seven objectives that were not met were cigarette use, smokeless tobacco use, binge drinking, illicit drug use, healthy weight, fruit intake, and vegetable intake. Of interest, the exercise and obesity objectives that were met are those where the military maintains strict performance standards, indicating that the military can achieve behavioral change within its organizational structure. However, without formal requirements or strong norms, it will be challenging to meet the targets for the other objectives because they involve choices around a number of behaviors that service members may not be motivated to make (e.g., not smoking, responsible drinking, having a proper diet).

Overweight (body mass index, or BMI $\geq$ 25) increased from 50 % in 1995 to 60 % in 2008, although the rate for 2008 was nearly identical to the rate for 2005, suggesting a possible leveling off of the increase. These increases are consistent with findings on overweight in the civilian population (Flegal, Carroll, Ogden, & Curtin, 2010), but are surprising in view of the emphasis on physical fitness in the military and suggest that other factors, such as dietary intake or genetic background, likely also play a role in overweight (Lindquist & Bray, 2001). Age, gender, and pay grade were among the strongest predictors of overweight: overweight was higher among persons aged 35 and older than among other age groups, higher among men than among women, and higher among enlisted personnel and warrant officers than among commissioned officers. The upward trend in overweight is disturbing regardless of the reasons for it, and it is a concern in that it likely reflects a reduction in the overall physical fitness of service members, which may compromise their ability to carry out their military mission. Military leaders will need to give additional attention to the factors that are contributing to the trend of increasing overweight and develop interventions to reverse it. The leveling off of the rate of overweight in 2008 from 2005 may indicate that a positive change has already begun, but this will need careful monitoring and additional vigorous efforts to reduce this trend.

In contrast to overweight, the rate of reported illnesses decreased notably from 1995 to 2008. This rate declined sharply (by over half) from 1995 to 1998 followed by stable rates in 2002 and 2005 and an increase in 2008, but it remained below the rate for 1995. It is encouraging to see the reduction in 1998, but it is unclear why the rate dropped so much or why it increased in 2008, although the latter may be related to the increase observed in injuries during this same period as summarized below. Of note, an injury that kept persons from work for a week or longer was the strongest predictor of illness. Service members with such an injury were 7.5 times more likely to report an illness than those without an injury. In addition, illness was higher among warrant officers and enlisted personnel than among commissioned officers, higher among those reporting high combat exposure than among those who had been deployed but had no combat exposure, and higher among women than among men. Personnel who used illicit drugs, who screened positive for anxiety, or who screened positive for PTSD were more likely to report illness than their counterparts. Clearly, the military environment, combat conditions, substance abuse choices, and mental health problems are all related to illness of service members and suggest the challenges that military leaders face in addressing the numerous variables that can affect the health of service members.

Similar to overweight, injuries showed an increase from 1995 to 2008. Rates were relatively low from 1995 to 2002 at 15 % followed by a steep increase to 39 % in 2005 and which held at that level in 2008. These higher injury rates for 2005 and 2008 are most likely due to increased tempo associated with training for combat or to war injuries from the conflicts in Iraq and Afghanistan during this period. The strong relationship between illness and injury noted above was further confirmed in our findings that illness was the strongest predictor of injury. Service members with an illness that kept them from duty for at least a week in the past year were over seven times more likely to report an injury than those without such an illness. Injury was also higher among persons aged 35 or older than among younger persons and lower among warrant officers than among those in other pay grades. In addition, injury was more likely among personnel with a history of physical or sexual abuse, among those who got less than 4 h of sleep a night, among those who screened positive for generalized anxiety disorder (GAD), and among illicit drug users.

Clearly, many factors increase risk for injuries, some of which may not seem obvious, but which require attention because injuries directly reduce force readiness and productivity. Indeed, other researchers have identified injuries as the single most significant medical impediment to military readiness (Jones, Amoroso, Canham, Weyandt, & Schmitt, 1999) and the largest health problem faced by the military (Jones, Canham-Chervak, & Sleet, 2010). A complex array of personal, environmental, physical, psychological, and behavioral factors increase risks for injury and have to be considered by military leaders, policymakers, and researchers as part of injury surveillance and prevention efforts.

7.2.3 Stress and Mental Health Problems

Chapter 5 investigated trends in prevalence rates for stress and mental health and the effects of a wide range of risk and protective factors for multiple screening measures, including work and family stress, depression, GAD, PTSD, and suicidal ideation, as well as receipt of mental health counseling. We noted a progressive decrease between 1988 and 2008 in the percentage of service members reporting "a lot" of work and family stress in their lives, which seems counterintuitive in time of war. Indeed, looking at stress among civilians reveals the expected pattern of a general increase in stress in recent years. Examining the sources of stress provides a possible explanation of this apparent contradiction. Whereas service members cited deployment and being away from family as increased sources of stress, civilians pointed to money, housing costs, and job stability as their major sources of increased stress (Clay, 2011). Interestingly, active duty service members are largely buffered from and do not experience these latter stressors to the same degree as civilians, suggesting that military and civilian stressors may be quite different. Although there may be many reasons why service members show a decline in stress, two plausible ones are (a) successful military efforts to mitigate stress through stress-reduction interventions or resilience training (Meredith et al., 2011) and (b) effective adapting to the stressors in their environment such that prior stressful events from earlier years now appear as more routine events (Bray et al., 2010).

Between 1995 and 2008, the percentage of military personnel who met screening criteria for needing further depression evaluation or who reported receiving mental health counseling increased, while the percentage of personnel who reported thinking about suicide when stressed was relatively stable. In the 2008 HRB survey, 19.8 % of personnel perceived a need for mental health counseling and a similar number (20 %) received care. This is in contrast to the 2002 HRB survey in which 18.7 % perceived a need for treatment but only 12.5 % received care. This suggests that the gap between the perceived need for treatment and receipt of treatment may be closing and that the military's efforts in recent years to reduce the stigma associated with receiving mental health counseling have at least partially succeeded. Nonetheless, a sizable portion of personnel still believe that receiving counseling may be detrimental to one's career, which likely leads to a continued reluctance to receive mental health counseling.

Among the large number of potential risk factors examined as predictors of mental health issues, two factors predicted all mental health outcomes (i.e., work and family stress, depression, GAD, PTSD, and suicidal ideation, as well as receipt of mental health counseling). These were use of avoidance coping mechanisms (including substance use) and high levels of work or family stress. Two other factors—getting less than 5 h of sleep on average and a history of physical or sexual abuse—were significant predictors of all mental health outcomes except for suicidal ideation. In addition, our findings indicated that of the few potentially protective factors examined, use of active coping strategies was the primary protective factor against negative mental health outcomes. Active coping was associated with all mental health outcomes except high stress and anxiety. Military personnel who implemented active coping strategies were less likely to have mental health problems, whereas those who espoused avoidance coping strategies were most likely to suffer from negative mental health consequences.

These findings about coping style need to be qualified by the fact that we were only able to ask limited questions about protective factors and did not include some important ones such as social support, which has been shown to be a buffer against mental health problems (e.g., Greenberg & Jones, 2011; James, Van Kampen, Miller, & Engdahl, 2013). Further, the relationship between stress and coping can be complex (even sometimes paradoxical) and needs to take into account respondents' interpretation of stressful events along with their assessment of the effectiveness of their coping strategies (Dolan & Ender, 2008),

7.2.4   Effects of Military and Psychosocial Factors

Throughout the analyses in this book, we have sought to consider the association of military and psychosocial factors, including deployment and combat exposure, with regard to our intermediate health and behavioral health outcomes of substance abuse, health, and mental health. Results showed that our measure of deployment and combat exposure was a significant predictor for any illicit drug use, heavy alcohol use, GAD, and PTSD in the past month. The finding that both non-deployment and high combat exposure were significantly associated with illness, injury, and the receipt of mental health counselling in the past year demonstrates the complexity of this bimodal relationship: those service members with mental health problems are likely coming into contact with the health care system either after heavy combat exposure or before they ever deploy. This suggests that pre-deployment screening may be working to prohibit or delay deployment for many with mental health problems and that post-deployment screening efforts may be missing some service members with mental health problems who have had moderate levels of combat exposure.

Another powerful predictor of our intermediate outcomes was high work or family stress. Those reporting high levels of work or family stress were more likely to be cigarette smokers, to report an injury in the past year, and to meet screening criteria for all of the mental health outcomes, including receipt of counselling.

Interestingly, high stress was protective for overweight/obesity, which is perhaps indicative of lack of appetite.

Past year injury and illness were the strongest predictors of one another as well as of illicit drug use, including prescribed medication misuse, GAD, and mental health counselling. Whereas illness alone was associated with PTSD, injury alone was associated with high stress and depression. These relationships are clearly intertwined and deserving of further research.

7.2.5   Productivity Loss Associated with Substance Use, Physical Health, and Mental Health

Chapter 6 examined the independent and combined effects on workforce productivity of substance abuse, physical health and health behaviors, and stress and mental health problems. We analyzed trends in productivity loss and developed a health and behavioral health model of productivity loss. Our final outcome workforce of productivity was measured in terms of past year self-reported productivity loss based on a 5-item scale assessing lowered work performance and absenteeism.

Our analysis of trends in overall productivity loss between 1995 and 2008 showed that although rates of productivity loss were relatively low among military personnel, they showed small but significant increases over time indicating that productivity decreased. Rates of productivity loss were higher among illicit drug users, heavy drinkers, and cigarette smokers compared with those who did not use these substances. Productivity loss was also related to more negative physical health behaviors. Service members who exercised regularly reported significantly less productivity loss than those who did not exercise regularly. Similarly, personnel who were overweight during the latter part of the period showed higher rates of productivity loss than their nonoverweight counterparts. Productivity loss was also related to mental health status. Personnel who reported high stress were more likely than those without high stress to experience productivity loss, and service members who screened positive for depression had significantly more productivity loss than those who did not meet criteria for depression. A key concern about productivity loss is the associated cost. Even seemingly small increases translate into significant monetary losses and reductions in overall readiness. For example, it is estimated that alcohol abuse alone cost DoD $745 million in reduced readiness and judicial expenses (e.g., prosecution of misconduct charges) in 2006 (Harwood, Zhang, Dall, Olaiya, & Fagan, 2009).

We also developed and estimated a health and behavioral health model of productivity loss that examined the impact of substance abuse, health and health behaviors, and mental health on productivity loss using a two-step process. In the first step, we estimated latent factors (i.e., inferred underlying measurement constructs using a set of observed variables) for substance use, mental health, and productivity loss. The analyses showed that each of the estimated latent factors provided a good fit for model estimation. Indicators for the substance use latent factor were alcohol dependence, one or more serious consequences of alcohol use, nicotine dependence, heavy drinking, past month smoking, and past month illicit drug use. Indicators for the mental health latent factor were PTSD, depression, GAD, significant work or family stress, receipt of mental health counseling services, and past year suicidal ideation. Indicators of the productivity loss latent factor were five items that examined the number of work days in the past year that service members reported working below their normal level of performance, being hurt in an on-the-job accident, coming to work late, leaving work early, or being absent from work.

In the second step, we entered a variety of variables into a path model that showed the relations between these variables and our measure of productivity loss. These consisted of the substance use and mental health latent factors along with three measures of physical health (overweight or obesity, illness in the past year, injury in the past year) and two single-item measures of activity limitations (poor physical health kept personnel from doing their usual activities, such as work or recreation; poor mental health kept personnel from doing their usual activities, such as work or recreation).

We included paths in the model to estimate the direct impact of substance use, mental health, and the three physical health items on productivity loss, as well as indirect pathways from these predictors through physical health- and mental health-related activity limitations. Together, the substance use and mental health latent constructs coupled with our measures of overweight/obesity, past year illness, past year injury, physical health limited usual activities, and mental health limited usual activities did a good job of predicting productivity loss. The model had an overall R^2 of 0.334, indicating that it explained one-third of the variance, which is relatively strong in a complex behavioral study such as this one.

The strongest predictor of productivity loss was activity limitations related to physical health. Mental health, injury, and illness were also strong predictors, while mental health-related activity limitations and substance use were significant but less strong predictors. These predictors showed direct effects on productivity loss and indicated that military personnel who reported physical limitations, injuries, or mental health problems were less able to be effective in their jobs and were more likely to work below normal performance levels, get hurt on the job, leave work early, or be late for or absent from work. This is consistent with other research showing that among both active duty and Reserve component personnel, service members with high stress and other mental health problems, as well as physical illness and injury, had greater productivity loss than those without these problems (Bray et al., 2009; Hourani et al., 2007; Hourani, Williams, & Kress, 2006).

Substance abuse had a direct but more moderate effect on productivity loss, potentially indicating an abuse pattern that may be more limited to times away from work such as evenings and weekends. In addition, the majority of indirect effects were significant, indicating that having more mental health problems and an injury or illness in the past year was associated with an increased likelihood of both mental health and physical health-related activity limitations predictive of productivity loss. That is, mental health, injury, and illness in the past year had an effect on productivity loss through both mental and physical health limitations of usual activities, indicating that productivity was negatively impacted by these problems both directly and indirectly. Service providers and policymakers should be alerted to this double impact, which underscores the importance of making mental health, injury, and illness a priority for improving readiness in the military, given the practical implications for DoD resources.

7.2.6   Study Limitations

Like all studies, ours had several limitations. All data were collected as part of the cross-sectional study design of the HRB surveys and therefore cannot be interpreted as being indicative of causal inference. We can learn much from the series of cross-sectional HRB surveys, but we acknowledge that relations among the variables that we examined are associations. We took steps to infer the most likely causal links where possible, but for any given survey year such as in our analyses from the 2008 survey in much of the book, it is not possible to determine conclusively which factors influenced which without a prospective approach. Additionally, these data represent only active duty forces; the total military force also includes National Guard and Reserve (NGR) and Coast Guard members, many of whom were mobilized and deployed in support of OIF/OEF as well as other combat and noncombat missions during this period. Similar data from NGR and Coast Guard personnel have been collected and analyzed elsewhere (Bray et al., 2011; Hourani et al., 2007; Lane, Hourani, Bray, & Williams, 2012).

As with all retrospective data, responses are as good as participants' memories and willingness to report accurate information. The fact that the HRB surveys were completed anonymously and several steps were taken to ensure pressure-free reporting helped to encourage the completion and accurate reporting of sometimes sensitive items. For example, the instrument was designed so that regardless of their answers, all participants would finish at approximately the same rate in the group administration survey setting. We ensured that all participation was voluntary and that no military personnel had access to completed survey data. Participants could skip any items they desired, and the instrument was held to a 30-page maximum to limit the amount of missing data while gathering the maximum amount of information.

Although many measures were standardized and almost all measures used in the questionnaires had been used in other national or military surveys, several measures (e.g., coping strategies, stress measures) lacked adequate psychometric information to determine reliability and/or validity in the active duty population. In addition, our measure of productivity loss was focused on behavioral or workforce productivity and did not include other potential indicators of productivity such as task speed and accuracy. However, because the concepts of productivity and productivity loss vary across industries and are especially difficult to define for the active duty military, we believe that the measures included here are valuable in uncovering previous relationships among substance abuse, physical health, and mental health issues in this population. Our findings hold potential for monitoring productivity loss as well as developing job-specific productivity measures that may be more relevant to particular job families within the military context.

A final limitation is that many of our analyses are drawn from data gathered in 2008 and are influenced by the historical events that were in play during that time, including the OIF/OEF armed conflicts. Although many of the issues facing the military today are similar to those in 2008 (e.g., recruiting, training, building cohesive units, supporting service members and families during deployments, reintegrating returning service members with their units and families), the specific challenges may change over time.

7.3   Programmatic Approaches to Improve Military Productivity

Although numerous programs exist within DoD and the Department of Veterans Affairs for service members returning from combat with substance abuse, health problems, or mental health problems, over the past several decades the military has implemented a number of additional efforts to improve the overall health and well-being of active duty military personnel and thereby improve military productivity. Indeed, both acute and long-term treatment and health promotion programs have grown in number and in scope, aiming to increase prevention and effective treatment of these types of problems among active duty, Reserve component, veterans, and family members. These problems persist as significant concerns for the military not only because of the immediate impacts to the individual, but also because of the cascading effect on the unit and the force overall in terms of readiness and productivity.

This sort of combined, multipronged approach that considers the overall health and well-being of military personnel is needed to address the multitude of factors that detract from military productivity and readiness. Preventing substance abuse is a cornerstone of *Healthy People 2020* objectives (Department of Health and Human Services & Office of Disease Prevention and Health Promotion, 2012) and military health promotion policy; equally important are the treatment, rehabilitation, and reintegration of substance abusers. DoD- and service-level campaigns seek to prevent alcohol abuse by increasing awareness about problems that can result from excessive drinking and encouraging responsible alcohol use (Bray, Brown, & Lane, 2013). These efforts include the DoD That Guy campaign, whose goal is to reduce excessive drinking among young servicemen (Department of Defense, 2013), and the Prime for Life program, which has been incorporated into substance abuse prevention and treatment frameworks across all branches of service. Prime for Life seeks to reduce the risk for health problems and impairment problems by increasing abstinence, delaying initial use, and decreasing high-risk use (Prevention Research Institute, 2013). However, many such programs lack sufficient evaluation of their efficacy in terms of both outcomes and cost, and are in need of ongoing expansion and updating.

The services also provide prevention and intervention resources for other substance use problems. Governed by Army Regulation 600-85, the Army Substance Abuse Program (ASAP) emphasizes readiness and personal responsibility in the prevention and treatment of substance abuse among the U.S. soldiers (Department of the Army, 2012a). Similarly, OPNAVINST 5350.4D (Department of the Navy, 2009) provides comprehensive alcohol and other drug abuse prevention and control policy and procedures for Navy and Marine Corps personnel, and establishes regulations to enforce this policy through the Navy Alcohol and Drug Abuse Prevention program (NADAP) and Substance Abuse Rehabilitation Program (SARP). The Air Force Alcohol and Drug Abuse Prevention and Treatment (ADAPT) program offers substance abuse treatment, referrals, and personnel training services, as well as family programs, testing programs, and civilian employee assistance (Military Health System, 2009).

Healthy and fit service members are critical to a ready military force, and as such physical health is another integral component of the *Healthy People 2020* objectives (Department of Health and Human Services & Office of Disease Prevention and Health Promotion, 2012). As noted in Chap. 4, lifestyle choices related to diet and exercise can have a positive or negative impact on health. All service members participate in routine physical fitness assessments and are scored against established performance criteria that are normed to age and gender. These criteria are designed to ensure that service members maintain good physical health and are conditioned to perform their military duties; personnel failing to meet these standards often engage in remedial physical training to heighten performance and enhance readiness. In addition to exercise and nutrition, illness and injuries are also of concern to military leadership because they negatively impact the readiness and productivity of the armed forces. DoD provides comprehensive health care at little or no cost to service members that comprise both health promotion (prevention of illness and injury) as well as treatment for issues that do arise. This dual approach is typically managed at the local installation clinic or hospital level, or, if needed, at major DoD medical centers.

In recent years, military leaders have placed increased emphasis on improving the resilience of service members, addressing mental health problems, the challenges of deployments and combat exposure, and have been making efforts to reduce the high rates of suicide among military personnel. Recognizing that combat-related behavioral health problems could not be adequately addressed by reactive efforts alone, the Army established the Directorate of Comprehensive Soldier Fitness (CSF) with the goal of increasing soldiers' resilience to stressful situations and combat environments. Based on recent work in the field of positive psychology, a resilience program was developed to provide soldiers with coping skills and techniques to strengthen psychological health (Adler, Bliese, & Castro, 2011; Department of the Army, 2012b). Both the Navy and Marine Corps established similar programs that incorporate resilience training with their Combat and Operational Stress Control (COSC) programs. An important aspect of the Marine Corps resilience program is the Operational Stress Control and Readiness (OSCAR) initiative to deliver mental health services to operating forces by embedding mental health professionals with deploying troops who are charged with educating before, during, and after deployment as well as treating combat stress injuries (Nash, 2006). The Air Force also developed its own resiliency program, which is part of the Deployment Transition Center. The purpose of this program is to allow airmen in selected missions some extra time to decompress and start to reintegrate back into day-to-day life (Department of the Air Force, 2010).

An important initiative to identify potentially avoidable risk factors for suicide is the Department of Defense Suicide Event Report (DODSER) Program, which mandates that comprehensive information regarding the background of personnel committing suicide be reported to the program within 30 days of the event. Together with research initiatives such as the Army Study to Assess Risk and Resilience in Servicemembers (STARRS), these programs hold promise for providing the data needed to propose policy changes that may reduce the risk of suicide.

In addition, the Defense Centers of Excellence for Psychological Health and Traumatic Brain Injury (DCoE) was established in 2007 "to integrate knowledge and identify, evaluate and disseminate evidence-based practices and standards for the treatment of psychological health and TBI within the Defense Department. DCoE works across the entire continuum of care to promote resilience, rehabilitation and reintegration for warriors, families and veterans with psychological health concerns and traumatic brain injuries" (http://www.dcoe.health.mil/WhatWeDo.aspx).

The approach that the military has taken to "stand up" new programs to address emerging needs of service members as they arise is impressive and shows the commitment the military continues to put forth to support and care for its members. A critical next step is to evaluate and determine whether or not these new efforts are effective and having their desired impact, with those shown to be efficacious being deployed on a widespread basis and those not shown to be efficacious being modified or eliminated from practice.

In the current climate of both great programmatic need and cost-effectiveness requirements, prevention will be the key. Two recent IOM reports—one on substance use disorders and the other on reintegration issues associated with returning home from OIF/OEF—both point to notable gaps and needed improvements in the DoD and Veterans Administration systems. They highlight needed research to address numerous unanswered questions and point to cultural changes that will be required to realize progress (IOM, 2012, 2013), noting that "culture change will require the use of strong prevention programs that use the full range of evidence-based prevention interventions" (IOM, 2012). The reports also recommended the development of strategies for identifying and diagnosing problems; providing treatment and rehabilitation; offering education outreach and community support programs; adopting, implementing, and disseminating evidence-based programs and best practices; increasing access to care; and strengthening the workforce (IOM, 2012, 2013).

These recommendations likely apply equally well to other military health behavior initiatives. Indeed, at least four recent publications echoed similar prevention and evidenced-based strategies in mental health applications and promotion (Adler et al., 2011; Department of the Army, 2012b; IOM, 2013; Kennedy & Zillmer, 2012). This book represents a significant step forward in providing key data needed for an evidence-based framework for program evaluation, which should include the evaluation of existing programs and the development, implementation, and evaluation of future programs as deemed necessary through the evaluation cycle.

7.4 Further Investigations

In this book, we purposely focused our analyses at the DoD level in which we aggregated information across personnel in the active duty Army, Navy, Marine Corps, and Air Force to provide a broad perspective for the active military. Although our approach has value, other analyses are needed to help understand the limits and applicability of these findings by applying them to different sectors and subpopulations within the military, such as for military men and women, for each of the military service branches, and for enlisted personnel and officers.

In addition, the applicability of these findings and models for the active duty population should be extended to the Reserve population using companion HRB data from the 2006 and 2010–2011 Surveys of Health Related Behaviors Among the Reserve Component. As the National Guard and Reserves have been increasingly called upon to help meet the needs of the military mission, they have experienced many of the same stressors and problems as their active duty counterparts, but it is unknown how and how well they deal with them. In addition, the Reserve component encounters problems that are distinctly associated with Reserve status such as arranging extended leaves of absence with civilian employers, planning for reintegration upon their return, and helping their families adjust to their variable work status (Lane et al., 2012). Combining current findings for the active component with analyses of these domains and models for the Reserve component would provide a comprehensive picture of the total military force.

Not surprisingly, our findings have raised new questions and suggest areas and issues that would benefit from additional careful investigation. Many of the analyses in this book point to the role of work and family stress and deployment and combat exposure on substance abuse, physical health problems, and mental health problems. Further investigations, particularly longitudinal studies, of personnel with repeated deployments, intense sources of stress at work and at home, and the weakness of avoidance coping mechanisms could improve our knowledge about these domains and ultimately about workforce productivity.

Our analyses have examined the effects of substance abuse, physical health, and mental health and assessed their effects on productivity loss. Within limits, we were able to assess their overlap, particularly among the mental health outcomes. However, further in-depth analyses and modeling approaches are needed that give greater attention to the comorbidities among the outcome measures across these three domains. Persons with comorbid substance abuse and mental health problems have been shown to have persistent functional impairment (Koenen et al., 2003; Wilk, Riviere, McGurk, Castro, & Hoge, 2010) and low rates of treatment (OAS, 2003). Comorbid mental health problems are also associated with somatic disorder, including metabolic syndrome (Jakovljevic, Saric, Nad, Topic, & Vuksan-Cusa, 2006), more physical symptoms (Hoge, Terhakopian, Castro, Messer, & Engel, 2007), and an increased illness burden (Campbell et al., 2007). Further research on these comorbidities could extend the recommendations of Falk, Yi, and Hilton (2008) to address the temporal ordering of all three of these domains, especially relative to deployment and/or combat/stress exposures, as well as to examine the range of personality issues that may increase vulnerability to the incidence and persistence of health-related problems among service members (Hasin & Kilcoyne, 2012).

Future studies should also expand the construct of productivity and its corollary, productivity loss. Our measure of productivity loss based on lower work performance and absenteeism has been informative, but future studies would benefit from broader measures of worker productivity such as the ability to meet peak performance demands, job satisfaction, and achievement of individual and military goals.

7.5   Concluding Comments

In this book, we have documented the prevalence, trends, and correlates across a variety of outcomes for the domains of substance abuse, physical health, and mental health based on data from 10 comprehensive HRB surveys spanning nearly 3 decades. We have also examined the impact of these domains on a health and behavioral health model of productivity loss. This book provides the first broad-based examination of the physical health and behavioral health of the active military force over time and shows how the health and behavior of our service members jointly impact their productivity and readiness. One of the key contributions of our study has been the ability through the richness of the HRB data to examine together the influence of an array of complex factors in these important cross-cutting domains.

The role of each of our domains in productivity loss suggests multiple prevention and intervention target points that are well-aligned with the emerging total force fitness paradigm championed by Admiral Mullen, the former Chair of the DoD Joint Chiefs of Staff (Mullen, 2010). If fully and carefully implemented, this paradigm will contribute to improved productivity of our service members in key ways spanning the lifecycle of military service. Improved screening of military recruits may help to identify existing problems with substance abuse, health, and mental health, or to predict the likelihood of developing these problems, so that individuals can be appropriately excluded from service or receive targeted prevention efforts according to their needs. Continued screening throughout the course of military service can lead to early detection and intervention for newly developed problems, allowing treatment to begin sooner and improving treatment trajectories (e.g., among combat veterans). Because our findings indicate that stress, mental health, and substance abuse all have significant negative impacts on productivity and readiness, additional training in evidence-based stress management techniques, coping strategies, and efforts to modify the culture of alcohol use should be considered as approaches that could help to stem the incidence of substance abuse and mental health problems and thus increase the productivity of the force.

Our findings about the strong connection of injury, mental health, and activity limitations to productivity loss provide key areas to target for improvements. Several efforts are underway to integrate technological advances, such as smartphones, virtual reality, and biofeedback, into screening, referral, prevention, and treatment processes within the military (e.g., Bernier, Bouchard, Robillard, Morin, & Forget, 2011; Hourani et al., 2011; Rizzo et al., 2011). These efforts show promise for engaging service members in monitoring their own physical and mental health and well-being, and therefore may be helpful in improving physical and mental health and reducing productivity loss.

Findings suggest that investing in worker health, including physical and mental health, in the form of both preventative efforts and treatment efforts, will improve productivity and personnel readiness. Sharing these data and research findings with service members and military leadership at all levels—including how substance abuse, physical health problems, and mental health problems jeopardize the ability to be the best service members and military force they can be—may help alleviate some of the stigma associated with seeking help in the military.

This book represents a significant step forward in providing the data needed for evidence-based program development. Continuing to identify and understand threats to the productivity of the military may help to create and maintain programs and policies that promote the high level of strength, energy, and focus required for current and future missions. We hope that our findings will generate interest from military leaders and policymakers and will lead to improvements in the quality of life for our service members and their families who collectively create the backbone of our military force.

References

Adler, A. B., Bliese, P. D., & Castro, C. A. (Eds.). (2011). *Deployment psychology*. Washington, DC: American Psychological Association.

Ames, G. M., Cunradi, C. B., Moore, R. S., & Stern, P. (2007). Military culture and drinking behavior among U.S. Navy careerists. *Journal of Studies on Alcohol and Drugs, 68*(3), 336–344.

Bernier, F., Bouchard, S., Robillard, G., Morin, B., & Forget, H. (2011). Enhancing stress management skills in military personnel using biofeedback and immersion in a stressful video-game: A randomized control trial. *Journal of Cybertherapy & Rehabilitation, 4*, 3.

Bray, R. M., Rae Olmsted, K. L., & Williams, J. (2012). Misuse of prescription pain medications in U.S. active duty service members. In: B. K. Wiederhold (Ed.), *Pain syndromes: From recruitment to returning troops: Vol. 91. NATO Science for Peace and Security Series E: Human and Societal Dynamics* (pp. 3–16). Amsterdam, Netherlands: IOS Press.

Bray, R. M., Brown, J. M., & Lane, M. E. (2013). Alcohol misuse prevention in the military. In: P. M. Miller (Ed.), *Interventions for addiction: Comprehensive addictive behaviors and disorders* (pp. 769–778). San Diego, CA: Elsevier.

Bray, R. M., Brown, J. M., & Williams, J. (2013). Trends in binge and heavy drinking and alcohol consumption-related problems: Implications of combat exposure in the U.S. Military. *Substance Use and Misuse, 48*(10), 799–810. doi:10.3109/10826084.2013.796990.

Bray, R. M., Pemberton, M. R., Hourani, L. L., Witt, M., Rae Olmsted, K. L., Brown, J. M., Weimer, B. J., Lane, M. E., Marsden, M. E., Scheffler, S. A., Vandermaas-Peeler, R., Aspinwall, K. R., Anderson, E. M., Spagnola, K., Close, K. L., Gratton, J. L., Calvin, S. L., & Bradshaw, M. R. (2009). *2008 Department of Defense survey of health related behaviors among active duty military personnel*. Report prepared for TRICARE Management Activity, Office of the

Assistant Secretary of Defense (Health Affairs) and U.S. Coast Guard. Research Triangle Park, NC: Research Triangle Institute.

Bray, R. M., Pemberton, M. R., Lane, M. E., Hourani, L. L., Mattiko, M. J., & Babeu, L. A. (2010). Substance use and mental health trends among U.S. military active duty personnel: Key findings from the 2008 DoD Health Behavior Survey. *Military Medicine, 175*(6), 390–399.

Bray, R. M., Rae Olmsted, K. L., Brown, J. M., Witt, M. B., Lane, M. E., Anderson, E. M., et al. (2011). *State of the behavioral health of the United States Coast Guard.* Research Triangle Park, NC: Research Triangle Institute.

Campbell, D. G., Felker, B. L., Liu, C. F., Yano, E. M., Kirchner, J. E., Chank, D., et al. (2007). Prevalence of depression-PTSD comorbidity: Implications for clinical practice guidelines and primary care-based interventions. *Journal of General Internal Medicine, 22*, 888–889.

Clay, R. A. (2011). Stressed in America. *Monitor on Psychology, 42*, 60–61.

Department of Defense. (2013). "That Guy" campaign website. Retrieved September 13, 2013, from http://www.thatguy.com

Department of Health and Human Services, Office of Disease Prevention and Health Promotion. (2012). *Healthy People 2020.* Washington, DC. Retrieved September 23, 2013, from http://www.healthypeople.gov/2020/default.aspx

Department of the Air Force. (2010). *Air Force Resiliency Program: Deployment transition center concept of operations.* Retrieved January 28, 2013, from http://www.ramstein.af.mil/shared/media/document/AFD-110103-001.pdf

Department of the Army. (2012a). Army Regulation 600-85, *The Army Substance Abuse Program.* Retrieved September 14, 2013, from http://www.apd.army.mil/pdffiles/r600_85.pdf

Department of the Army. (2012b). *Army 2020: Generating health and discipline in the force ahead of the strategic reset.* Washington, DC: Department of the Army.

Department of the Navy. (2009). OPNAVINST 5350.4D, *Navy alcohol and drug abuse prevention and control.* Retrieved September 13, 2013, from http://www.med.navy.mil/sites/nhoh/SiteCollectionDocuments/DAPA_5350_4D1.pdf

Dolan, C., & Ender, M. (2008). The coping paradox: Work, stress, and coping in the U.S. army. *Military Psychology, 20*, 151–169.

Falk, D. E., Yi, H. Y., & Hilton, M. E. (2008). Age of onset and temporal sequencing of lifetime DSM-IV alcohol use disorder relative to comorbid mood and anxiety disorders. *Drug and Alcohol Dependence, 94*, 234–245.

Flegal, K. M., Carroll, M. D., Ogden, C. L., & Curtin, L. R. (2010). Prevalence and trends in obesity among U.S. adults, 1999–2008. *Journal of the American Medical Association, 303*(3), 235–241.

Greenberg, N., & Jones, N. (2011). Optimizing mental health support in the military: The role of peers and leaders. In A. B. Adler, P. D. Bliese, & C. A. Castro (Eds.), *Deployment psychology.* Washington, DC: American Psychological Association.

Harris, K. M., & Edlund, M. J. (2005). Self-medication of mental health problems: New evidence from a national survey. *Health Services Research, 40*, 117–134.

Harwood, H. J., Zhang, Y., Dall, T. M., Olaiya, S. T., & Fagan, N. K. (2009). Economic implications of reduced binge drinking among the military health system's TRICARE Prime plan beneficiaries. *Military Medicine, 174*, 728–736.

Hasin, D., & Kilcoyne, B. (2012). Comorbidity of psychiatric and substance use disorder in the United States: Current issues and findings from the NESARC. *Current Opinion in Psychiatry, 25*, 165–171.

Hoge, C. W., Terhakopian, A., Castro, C. A., Messer, S. C., & Engel, C. C. (2007). Association of posttraumatic stress disorder with somatic symptoms, healthcare visits, and absenteeism among Iraq war veterans. *American Journal of Psychiatry, 164*, 150–153.

Hourani, L. L., Bray, R. M., Marsden, M. E., Witt, M., Vandermaas-Peeler, R, Schleffler, S., et al. (2007). *2006 Department of Defense survey of health related behaviors in the Reserve Component.* Report prepared for the U.S. Department of Defense (Cooperative Agreement No. DAMD17-00-2-0057).

Hourani, L. L., Kizakevich, P. N., Hubal, R., Spira, J., Strange, L. B., Holiday, D. B., et al. (2011). Predeployment stress inoculation training for primary prevention of combat-related stress disorders. *Journal of Cybertherapy & Rehabilitation, 4*, 101–116.

Hourani, L. L., Williams, T. V., & Kress, A. M. (2006). Stress, mental health, and job performance among active duty military personnel: Findings from the 2002 Department of Defense Health related Behaviors Survey. *Military Medicine, 171*(9), 849–856.

Institute of Medicine (IOM). (2012). *Substance use disorders in the U.S. armed forces.* Washington, DC: The National Academies Press.

Institute of Medicine (IOM). (2013). *Assessment of readjustment needs of veterans, service members, and their families.* Washington, DC: The National Academies Press.

Jacobson, I. G., Ryan, M. A. K., Hooper, T. I., Smith, T. C., Amoroso, P. J., Boyko, E. J., et al. (2008). Alcohol use and alcohol-related problems before and after military combat deployment. *Journal of the American Medical Association, 300*(6), 663–675.

Jakovljevic, M., Saric, M., Nad, S., Topic, R., & Vuksan-Cusa, B. (2006). Metabolic syndrome, somatic and psychiatric comorbidity in war veterans with post-traumatic stress disorder: Preliminary findings. *Psychiatria Danubia, 18*, 169–176.

James, L. M., Van Kampen, E., Miller, R. D., & Engdahl, B. E. (2013). Risk and protective factors associated with symptoms of post-traumatic stress, depression, and alcohol misuses in OEF/OIF veterans. *Military Medicine, 178*(2), 159–165.

Jonas, W. B., O'Connor, F. G., Deuster, P., Peck, J., Shake, C., & Frost, S. S. (2010). Why total force fitness? *Military Medicine, 175*(8), 6–13.

Jones, B. H., Amoroso, P. J., Canham, M. L., Weyandt, M. B., & Schmitt, J. B. (Eds.). (1999). Atlas of injuries in the U.S. armed forces. *Military Medicine, Supplement, 164*(8), S1–S633.

Jones, B. H., Canham-Chervak, M., & Sleet, D. A. (2010). An evidence-based public health approach to injury priorities and prevention: Recommendations for the U.S. *Military American Journal of Preventive Medicine, 38*(1 Suppl), S1–S10.

Kennedy, C. H., & Zillmer, E. A. (2012). *Military psychology: Clinical and operational applications* (2nd ed.). New York: The Guilford Press.

Koenen, K. C., Lyons, M. J., Goldberg, J., Simpson, J., Williams, W. M., Toomey, R., et al. (2003). Co-twin control study of relationships among combat exposure, combat-related PTSD and other mental disorder. *Journal of Traumatic Stress, 16*, 433–438.

Lane, M. E., Hourani, L. L., Bray, R. M., & Williams, J. (2012). Prevalence of perceived stress and mental health indicators among Reserve Component and active duty military personnel. *American Journal of Public Health, 102*, 1213–1220.

Lindquist, C. H., & Bray, R. M. (2001). Trends in overweight and physical activity among US military personnel, 1995–1998. *Preventive Medicine, 32*(1), 57–65.

Meredith, L. S., Sherbourne, C. D., Gaillot, S., Hansell, L., Ritschard, H. V., Parker, A. M., et al. (2011). *Promoting psychological resilience in the U.S. military.* Arlington: Rand Center for Military Health Policy Research.

Military Health System. (2009). *Department of Defense survey of health related behaviors among active duty military personnel: Service program offerings.* Retrieved September 13, 2013, from http://tricare.mil/tma/dhcape/surveys/coresurveys/surveyhealthrelatedbehaviors/downloads/FINALHBProgramSheet_Feb2010.pdf

Mullen, M. (2010). On total force fitness in war and peace. *Military Medicine, 175*(8), 1–2.

Nash, W. P. (2006) Operational Stress Control and Readiness (OSCAR): The United States Marine Corps Initiative to Deliver Mental Health Services to Operating Forces. In *Human dimensions in military operations: military leaders' strategies for addressing stress and psychological support* (pp. 25-1–25-10). Meeting Proceedings RTO-MP-HFM-134, Paper 25. Neuilly-sur-Seine, France: RTO.

Office of Applied Studies. (2003). *Results from the 2002 National Survey on drug use and health: Summary of national findings* (DHHS Publication No. SMA 03-3836, NSDUH series H-ss). Rockville, MC: Substance Abuse and Mental health Services Administration.

Prevention Research Institute. (2013). *Prime for life*. Lexington, KY: Author. Retrieved September 13, 2013, from http://www.primeforlife.org/homepage.cfm

Rizzo, A., Parsons, T. D., Lange, B., Kenny, P., Buckwalter, J. G., Rothbaum, B., et al. (2011). Virtual reality goes to war: A brief review of the future of military behavioral healthcare. *Journal of Clinical Psychology in Medical Settings, 18*(2), 176–187.

Smith, T. C., Zamorski, M., Smith, B., Riddle, J., WeardMann, C. A., Wells, T. S., et al. (2007). The physical and mental health of a large military cohort: Baseline functional health status of the Millennium Cohort. *BMC Public Health, 7*, 340.

Tanielian, T., & Jaycox, L. H. (2008). *Invisible Wounds of War: Psychological and Cognitive Injuries, their Consequences, and Services to Assist Recovery*. Santa Monica, CA: Center for Military Health Policy Research, Rand Corporation.

Wilk, T., Riviere, L. A., McGurk, D., Castro, C. A., & Hoge, C. W. (2010). Prevalence of mental health problems and functional impairment among active component and National Guard soldiers 3 and 12 months following combat in Iraq. *Archives of General Psychiatry, 67*, 614–623.

Williams, J. O., Bell, N. S., & Amoroso, P. J. (2002). Drinking and other risk taking behaviors of enlisted male soldiers in the US Army. *Work, 18*, 141–150.

Index

R.M. Bray et al., *Understanding Military Workforce Productivity: Effects of Substance Abuse, Health, and Mental Health*, DOI 10.1007/978-0-387-78303-1, © Springer Science+Business Media New York 2014